FIRST AID AND HEALTH CARE FOR DOGS

Charles T.P. Bell
M.A. Vet. M.B., MRCVS

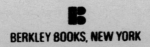

BERKLEY BOOKS, NEW YORK

This Berkley book contains the complete
text of the original edition.

FIRST AID AND HEALTH CARE FOR DOGS

A Berkley Book / published by arrangement with
Pecos Press

PRINTING HISTORY
Pecos Press edition published 1990
Berkley edition / June 1991

ISBN: 0-425-13129-7

A BERKLEY BOOK ® TM 757,375
Berkley Books are published by The Berkley Publishing Group,
200 Madison Avenue, New York, New York 10016.
The name "BERKLEY" and the "B" logo
are trademarks belonging to Berkley Publishing Corporation.

PRINTED IN THE UNITED STATES OF AMERICA

10 9 8 7

Contents

Medicating the Ears

Preface

It is my wish that no animal ever be confronted with a "life or death" situation. However, accidents do happen all too frequently. If your dog does suffer an injury, you must make several decisions in a very short period of time. Often, your choices will affect your pet's overall well-being. *First Aid & Health Care for Dogs* was written to help you make the right decisions.

No book can take the place of your veterinarian. In the time of a crisis, the best chance for a favorable outcome is to get your dog to your veterinarian as quickly as possible. You should not waste time trying to diagnose or to treat your pet's injury. However, there are some basic steps that you can take that might stabilize the animal, reducing the chance of further damage and complications. These are the procedures advocated in this book.

First Aid & Health Care for Dogs works as a bridge between your veterinarian and you. The two of you are partners that share the same goal: maintaining the good health of your dog. Reaching this goal is the best way to ensure that your dog will enjoy a long, happy life. The book can also help prepare you to make the right choices for decisions that, hopefully, you will never have to make.

The book is divided into three parts.

Part I–Health Care

Part I outlines the various components of a
   general health care program. These
   components are important to the maintenance of the overall good health of
   your dog. A healthy dog is in the best
   position to fight off diseases and the
   effects of injuries. In addition, proper
   health care for your pet will reduce the
   chance of the animal transmitting a
   parasite or disease to other members of
   your family.

Part II–First Aid

This section gives the first aid procedures
   that should be taken in many of the
   most common emergency situations.
   The steps described emphasize common sense, simplicity and your own
   safety.

Each chapter begins with a short overview
   that gives background information
   about the emergency. Next are the
   common signs that you are likely to see.
   These are followed by the proper steps
   to take. Just as important as telling you
   what to do, the book indicates what you
   should NOT do; it informs you of the
   common mistakes that people often
   make. Most chapters end by advising
   you to take your injured pet to your

veterinarian; Chapter 21 details the correct manner to do this.

The layout of each chapter facilitates quick and easy use. In the time of a crisis, you will not have to waste time searching for the proper steps to take.

Part III–After the Emergency

Your veterinarian may ask you to take an active role on the recuperative process. This section instructs you how to administer medicine, check devices used for healing and deal with various issues associated with surgery. The last chapter covers rehabilitation; it recommends steps to take that will help your dog regain its strength gradually and safely.

Writing a book is a difficult task. Without the help and guidance of many individuals, this project would not have been completed. I would like to thank all of the reviewers (both the veterinarians and the non-veterinarians) for their comments. They forced me to factor out my own medical biases as well as to keep the material readily accessible to the intended audience. A special debt of gratitude goes to Alice Dworkin, whose advice pointed me in the right direction and comments kept me on course throughout the project.

I would also like to thank A. Christine MacMurray, Editor at the Animal Medical Center in New York City, for allowing me to access the the AMC's library while researching the material.

Lastly, Karen Fortgang of bookworks deserves credit for patiently guiding me through the various stages of production.

I would like to close with a word of warning. An injured animal can be a dangerous animal. A dog in pain may resist any handling and may try to bite you. You must be on guard and take precautions to protect yourself. If you are bitten, you should seek medical attention.

About the Author

Charles T. P. Bell graduated from Cambridge University with a degree in Veterinary Medicine. Dr. Bell has practiced for several years in both the United Kingdom and the United States, specializing in small animals.

PART I

HEALTH CARE

1 Preventive Medicine

Introduction

Preventive medicine is taking steps to prevent illness. By following a complete program, you help your dog maintain good health throughout its life. The most important aspects of a preventive medicine program are a well-balanced diet and regular veterinary examinations. Chapter 2 discusses nutrition (see page 21). Other components of preventive medicine are outlined below.

Going to Your Veterinarian

Regular trips to your veterinarian are crucial to the maintenance of your dog's health. Your doctor can design a program geared specifically for your dog. Periodic examinations will allow the veterinarian to monitor your dog's progress and adjust the program as needed. In addition, the veterinarian will know of special issues that apply to your geographic location (such as the length of flea and tick season, the prevalence of certain diseases and the local ordinances that pertain to pets).

You should visit your veterinarian for a number of reasons.

> • It is easier to prevent a disease than to treat it. Your dog is better off if steps are taken to prevent an illness rather than if steps are needed to treat one.

Some diseases cannot be treated (rabies being the most notorious).

- It is less expensive to prevent a disease than to treat it. Vaccinations may seem expensive, but they are much cheaper than a cure for an illness. The money spent on preventive medicine is like buying insurance against disease; it is the best insurance policy available for your pet.

- Your dog may not be the only one who gets sick. Some of the diseases that threaten your dog can be transmitted to humans. Taking steps to keep your dog disease-free is important to the overall health of the entire family.

Your first trip to your veterinarian should be soon after obtaining your dog or puppy. This is the best time to begin a complete health program. After the first series of visits, your dog should be examined by your veterinarian at least once each year. In addition, you should have a test for worms performed every 6 months to 1 year, depending on your area.

When Going to Your Veterinarian

- Take a recent fecal sample (also known as a stool sample). It should be less than 24 hours old; it will be used to check for worms and other intestinal parasites.
- Bring a leash. There will probably be sev-

eral other animals at the clinic. You must be able to keep your pet under control.

• Try to remember any recent unusual behavior exhibited by your dog. Give the veterinarian as many details as you can.

Vaccinations

Vaccinations are powerful tools that stimulate the immune system, the natural line of defense against disease. Once a virus or bacteria has been introduced and fought off, the immune system remembers it and develops a mechanism to fight it in the future. A vaccine is made from the same agent that causes a disease, but the agent is altered so that it is harmless. The immune system, however, cannot tell the difference between the real agent and the vaccine. This allows the system to build up a defense to the disease without being subjected to it.

Most vaccinations are given when your dog is young. Puppies should receive 2 to 4 shots a few weeks apart. Staging the shots allows your puppy to gradually build up adequate immunity. Until it has received all of them, your puppy may not be fully protected. Annual booster shots are needed to keep the immune system strong.

Diseases Prevented by Vaccinations

• Rabies—This is one of the most feared diseases; there is no cure. Rabies attacks the brain and the nervous system. The most common way that rabies is transmitted is through bites from infected wild animals. These often are raccoons, foxes, skunks, bats and stray dogs and cats.

Your puppy should have its first rabies vaccination at the age of 3 months. After that, the vaccination can be given once a year or every 3 years. Your veterinarian will advise you on the best vaccine for your dog.

If your dog is bitten by an animal that you suspect may have rabies, go to your veterinarian immediately. Your dog may need an additional booster shot to strengthen the immune system and may need to be quarantined for observation.

People can also contract rabies. Anyone bitten by an animal should seek medical attention immediately.

• Distemper—This attacks the respiratory, gastrointestinal and nervous systems. This disease can cause coughing, conjunctivitis, vomiting, diarrhea and dehydration. Despite treatment, it frequently results in death.

The distemper shot contains several

additional vaccines designed to stave off a variety of other diseases. These diseases are listed below.

- Parvovirus—A viral disease that causes severe vomiting and diarrhea containing blood. It leads to dehydration and can affect the heart muscle. Parvovirus is difficult to treat and frequently fatal.

- Leptospirosis—There are two types of this disease; both are bacterial and attack the kidneys, liver and red blood cells. They can be transmitted to people.

- Canine Hepatitis—A viral disease that attacks the liver. It causes jaundice, vomiting, diarrhea and dehydration. It is often fatal.

- Canine Parainfluenza—A viral disease that affects the respiratory system. It is rarely fatal but can be debilitating. It can cause a persistent infection that can lower the resistance of the immune system. This, in turn, makes the dog more susceptible to secondary respiratory infection which can be more serious.

- Corona Virus—This is a viral disease affecting the gastrointestinal tract. It can cause vomiting and diarrhea, often with both containing blood. This disease can lead to dehydration and can be fatal.

- Bordetella—Also known as Kennel Cough. It is a bacterial disease affecting the respiratory system. It is rarely fatal but can debilitate the dog for several weeks. The animal may have a hacking cough that often brings up a great deal of phlegm. During this time, the dog may be susceptible to secondary disease.

Neutering

Neutering is the removal of the reproductive glands, preventing a dog from breeding. While this helps control the dog population, it has medical and behavioral benefits as well. Neutering does not alter the personality of your dog.

- Males—Neutering for males is known as altering or castration; it is the removal of the testicles. The most common time to have a male altered is between the ages of 6 and 12 months.

Advantages of Altering

- Prevents unwanted pregnancies and puppies
- Often causes dog to be less aggressive (less likely to fight)
- Less likely to wander off (reducing its chance of being hit by car)
- Less likely to have prostate problems as it grows old

Disadvantages of Altering

- Cannot breed
- Has to have an operation requiring anesthesia
- Tends to gain weight (easily controlled by adjusting diet)

- Females—Neutering for females is known as spaying. This is the removal of the ovaries and uterus. The most common time to have a female spayed is between the ages of 6 and 12 months old.

Advantages of Spaying

- Prevents unwanted pregnancies and puppies
- Prevents bleeding during times in heat
- Greatly reduces the risk of breast

cancer, if performed early in life
- Eliminates the risk of pyometra (a very serious disease that involves the production of pus in the uterus).

Disadvantage of Spaying

- Cannot breed
- Has to have an operation requiring anesthesia
- Tends to gain weight (easily controlled by adjusting diet)

Unless you plan to breed your dog, you should elect to have it neutered. The risk is very low (especially for a young dog) and outweighed by the medical benefits.

Parasites

There are a number of parasites that can affect your dog. These include heartworm, worms, fleas, ticks, mites and mange. They are discussed in Chapter 3 (see page 31).

Exercise

Regular exercise promotes good health. It strengthens the muscles and causes the heart to pump blood throughout the body at a higher rate than normal. This aids the function of all of the internal organs and can reduce the chance of serious disease, such as heart disease and diabetes. Exercise burns up excess calories and helps prevent obesity. It is also fun for the dog and can stop many behavioral problems resulting from boredom, such as chewing on furniture and licking itself raw.

Exercise requirements vary greatly between dogs. Factors to take into consideration are the age of the dog, its size and the type of breed. A small dog kept in the home will need less exercise than a large athletic animal. Athletic dogs, such as working and hunting breeds, thrive on a great deal of exercise. This requires a large block of time on your part each day. You should take these factors into account when selecting a pet.

The best approach to exercise is to be both regular and even. Dogs should be exercised twice a day. "Even" exercise means a consistent amount and type of exercise over a period of time. To abruptly go from light to strenuous exercise can result in muscle damage or ligament and tendon strain. The type of exercise should be varied every so often to keep it from becoming too routine. This can prevent boredom for both the dog and you.

Skin Care

Good skin care helps prevent skin infections. These are usually difficult to treat and can lead to additional problems if a dog constantly bites or scratches itself. Once a dog has had a skin problem, it is often prone to contracting another.

- Brushing—Good skin care begins with daily brushing. This stimulates the skin, removes dead hair and dandruff, and prevents knots and mats from developing (especially on long-haired dogs). In addition, it allows you to closely examine your pet every day.

- Baths—Most dogs should be bathed every 6 months. Breeds that have greasy and excessively oily coats should be bathed more often, sometimes as often as every 2 to 4 weeks. Use a shampoo designed for dogs. (Human shampoos are too strong and can irritate the skin.)

- Diet Supplements—There are several food supplements that can aid your dog's skin. They may also help to make the coat shiny. Oversupplementation can be harmful; check with your veterinarian before beginning to use a supplement. Some suggestions are listed below.

  - Vitamins that have zinc
  - Eggs (once or twice a week)
  - Oils such as olive oil or corn oil. 1 to 3 teaspoons a day can be mixed into food. (This is for dogs with very dry skin.)

- Fleas—Fleas should be treated quickly.
  They cause the dog to scratch and can
  lead to skin infection. Fleas are discussed in greater detail in Chapter 3
  (see page 37).

Care of Teeth and Gums

The care of teeth and gums is increasingly recog-
nized as important for general good health. Dogs
with dental problems may develop bad breath and
may go off their food. Poor dental care may lead to
inflamed and infected gums, which can result in the
loss of teeth. There is a chance that an infection will
enter the bloodstream where it may affect internal
organs such as the kidneys. Bad teeth and gums are
especially debilitating for older animals. Consult
with your veterinarian as to what steps you should
take to foster strong teeth and gums. Some ideas
are discussed below.

- Giving bones—Marrow bones are extremely hard and are good for dental
  care. Chewing on a bone will help clean
  teeth and stimulate the gums. However, bones are not digestible. If one is
  swallowed, it may cause stomach and
  intestinal problems; in addition, the
  bone might have to be removed surgi-
  cally.

  Chicken and poultry bones splinter and
  break easily. They often get caught in
  the throat. These bones should never

be given to a dog.

- Giving rawhide—Rawhide can clean the teeth and stimulate the gums, just like marrow bones. But rawhide is digestible. Swallowing top-quality rawhide is rarely unhealthy.

- Giving biscuits—These are good treats; their hard texture helps take care of teeth and gums. They are easily digestible and often contain vitamins. However, do not give too many biscuits to your dog. Their calories may lead to a weight problem.

- Brushing teeth—Brushing your dog's teeth once a week is recommended. You should only use a toothbrush and toothpaste that are designed specifically for dogs; several products are available.

- Scraping off plaque—Plaque is a yellow film that forms on a tooth, usually where the gum and tooth meet. If you catch it early, you might be able to use a fingernail and scrape the plaque off. If not, removing the plaque may require heavy scraping with a special tool and an anesthetic. Do not be alarmed if scraping off plaque causes the gums to bleed a little. (Use caution so that you are not bitten; if your dogs does bite you, seek medical attention immediately.)

To Scrape Off Plaque

- Open dog's mouth.
- Place tip of fingernail on tooth to be scraped, right at the line where the gum and tooth meet.
- Gently push your fingernail under the gum line a little.

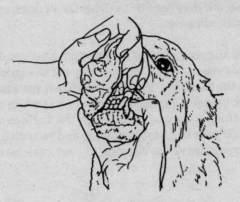

- Firmly scrape tooth in direction away from the gum.

Cleaning the Ears

Some breeds (such as spaniels and poodles) as well as individual dogs from all breeds are prone to ear infections. These dogs should have their ears periodically cleaned of excess hair and wax. Cleaning an ear is similar to administering ear medication (see page 151). Your veterinarian can recommend how often your dog's ears should be cleaned.

Clipping the Toenails

Your dog's toenails should not be allowed to grow too long. The proper length is such that the end of the toenail just meets the ground when your dog is standing naturally. Some dogs rarely need to have their nails clipped; walking on hard surfaces such as sidewalks, streets and playgrounds can file down the nails if they become too long. Other dogs require periodic clipping.

When clipping a nail, it is important that you do not cut too much. If you do, you may cut the quick, an area that consists of nerves and blood vessels. The quick is easily identified if the dog has white nails: it is the pink area just beneath the surface of the nail. (If your dog has black nails and you cannot see the quick, leave the clipping to your veterinarian.)

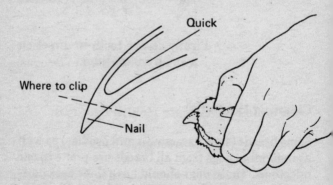

You should use a clipper especially designed for cutting the toenails of dogs. If you should accidently cut the quick and draw blood, take a wad of cloth or cotton and apply it directly to the bleeding nail. Hold it in place until the bleeding stops.

Impacted Anal Glands

If your dog is scraping its rear end along the ground, this is probably due to the impaction of the two anal glands. These glands are situated at the opening of the anus and secrete an aromatic fluid that is probably used to mark territory. Each gland has only one duct; as a result, the glands can easily be blocked. As pressure builds, they will begin to itch, causing the dog to try to alleviate the irritation.

Signs of Impacted Anal Glands

- Scraping, scooting or dragging its rear end along the ground
- Trying to relieve an itch around the anus

What to Do

- Transport to your veterinarian (see page 135).

Example of Complete Health Program

This is an example of a complete health program for a dog. Many variables need to factored into this program. These include type of dog, climate, local laws, and other regional issues. These factors can change from time to time. As such, your veterinarian is in the best position to design a program that is suited to the specific needs of your dog. The two of you should set up a program.

Puppy

- Soon after acquisition
    - Complete physical by your veterinarian

- 6 to 8 weeks
    - Distemper vaccination
    - Corona vaccination
    - Bordetella vaccination
    - Fecal test
    - Worming
    - Heartworm prevention program

- 10 to 12 weeks
    - Distemper vaccination
    - Corona vaccination
    - Bordetella vaccination
    - Rabies vaccination
    - Worming

- 14 to 16 weeks
    - Distemper vaccination
    - Corona vaccination
    - Bordetella vaccination

Adult

- Daily
    - Brush coat
    - Supplement food
    - Give heartworm pills (if using

daily medication)
- Give rawhide for teeth and gums

- **Weekly**
  - Brush teeth
  - Clean ears (if necessary)
  - Bathe with medicated shampoo (if necessary)

- **Monthly**
  - Give heartworm pills (if using monthly medication)
  - Bathe with medicated shampoo (if necessary)

- **6 Months**
  - Heartworm test (if heartworm is a year-round risk)
  - Fecal test
  - Worming
  - Bathe with medicated shampoo

- **Yearly**
  - General exam by your veterinarian
  - Rabies vaccination
  - Distemper vaccination
  - Corona vaccination
  - Bordetella vaccination
  - Heartworm test
  - Fecal test
  - Worming
  - Geriatric work-up (for older dog only)

Summary

- Preventive medicine is a crucial concern for the health of not only your dog but also your entire family.
- You should visit your veterinarian soon after acquiring your puppy or dog.
- The veterinarian should examine your dog at least once a year.
- Vaccinations help the immune system to fight off various diseases.
- Unless you plan to breed your dog, you should have it altered or spayed.
- Good skin care keeps the coat shiny and helps reduce shedding.
- Care of teeth and gums is an essential part of preventive medicine.

2 Nutrition

Introduction

Excellent health begins with good nutrition. The keys to good nutrition are plenty of fresh water and a well-balanced diet consisting of high quality food.

Fresh Water

It is crucial that your dog always has access to clean, fresh water. Lack of water can lead to dehydration. This can cause a wide variety of problems. It is a good idea to make water constantly available to your dog and to change the water daily. Adequate water is especially important for puppies and older dogs.

What to Feed

A well-balanced diet begins with the correct food. It is best to use a quality commercial diet which can be bought at supermarkets, at pet stores and from your veterinarian. Commercial food companies have spent years and millions of dollars on the perfection of their products. The result is that these foods provide the best mix of nutrients and flavor. A home-made diet can be well-balanced but it will probably be more expensive than a good commercial food and it may leave out important nutrients.

Once you have decided on a type of food, do not change very often. A dog's digestive system does not adapt well to sudden changes. Changing the type of food may upset the system, often causing vomiting and diarrhea.

It is important to clean the water and feed bowls on a regular basis. Also food must be stored properly after it has been opened; instructions for this are usually written on the package. Any food that appears moldy or has a rancid odor should be discarded.

Types of Food Available

There are four main types of dog food available today.

- Dry (cereal)
    - Low moisture; stays fresh in feed bowl
    - Inexpensive
    - Convenient
    - Least palatable and digestible
- Semi-Moist (cereal with some meat texture)
    - Stays fresh in feed bowl for several hours
    - Convenient
    - Moderately inexpensive
    - Moderately palatable and digestible
- Canned Ration (meat with cereal added)
    - Moderate cost
    - Moderately palatable and digestible

- Canned Meat (all meat)
    - Most nutritious, palatable and digestible
    - Most expensive
    - Spoils quickly; will not stay fresh in feed bowl

Several factors should be considered when selecting the best food for your dog. A few are listed below.

- Type of dog
    - Large, medium or small
    - Reputation of breed
    - Will eat any food or very finicky
- Age of dog
    - Puppy
    - Adult
    - Old
- Level of activity
    - House pet or working dog
    - Amount of daily exercise
- Environment
    - City or country
    - House or apartment
    - Size of home
    - Yard or no yard
    - One dog or more than one
- Cost of food

Special Diets

There are special diets available to assist in the treatment or management of important medical conditions, such as kidney disease, heart disease, obesity and several others. Your veterinarian can determine if your dog has a condition that may respond to dietary modification and can recommend the best product. While many "lite" foods are available to help promote weight loss, you should not make a change in diet without first consulting with your doctor.

How Much to Feed

Most dog foods have a feeding chart printed on the package. However, this chart should be used only as a rough guideline. Each dog is different; some need more food than others. By experimenting with various portions of food, you will eventually determine the best amount for your dog. Your veterinarian should be consulted on this matter, as well.

How Often to Feed

A guideline for how often to feed is below. Again, not all dogs are the same. Your veterinarian can help you determine the proper feeding schedule.

- Up to 3 months—4 times a day
- 3 to 4 months—3 times a day
- 4 to 6 months—2 times a day
- 6 months and beyond—once a day

Some adult dogs do better on 2 feedings. If you feed an adult dog twice a day, be careful not to overfeed it.

Controlling Weight

Ideal weight varies for each dog. Your veterinarian can help you determine the best weight for your dog. Once this has been established, you can help your dog maintain that weight through periodic evaluations. Three methods are outlined below.

Measuring by Sight

- Stand the dog up.
- Look at area between front legs and back legs.
- Dog is underweight if you can see each individual rib.
- Dog is overweight if you cannot tell where the rib cage ends and the abdominal area begins.
- Dog is at the ideal weight if there is good definition between the rib cage and the abdominal area.

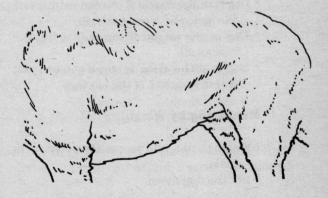

Measuring by Touch

- Stand the dog up.
- Place hands on opposite sides of the rib cage.

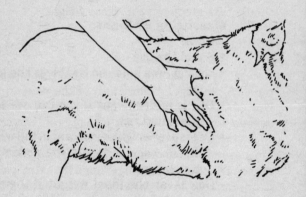

- Dog is underweight if you can readily feel the space between each rib.
- Dog is overweight if you cannot feel the ribs at all.
- Dog is at the ideal weight if you can just feel the outline of the rib cage.

Measuring by Weighing

- Weigh the dog and yourself on a bathroom scale.
- Set the dog down.

- Weigh yourself alone.
- Subtract your weight from that of the dog and you combined. The difference is the weight of the dog.

If your dog is underweight, you should increase its daily amount of food. If your dog is overweight, you should take steps to help it lose weight.

Losing Weight

Excess weight is the most common nutritional problem for dogs. Almost half of the dogs in the United States suffer from obesity. An overweight dog is a walking time bomb. Obesity contributes to such serious long-term illnesses as heart disease, hip degeneration, diabetes and certain forms of cancer. In addition, lugging around the extra weight is uncomfortable (especially in hot weather). You can help your dog lose weight.

Steps for Weight Loss

- Reduce amount of food given per day by a third.
- Change regular food to a special diet food.
- Eliminate all snacks.
- Increase the amount of daily exercise.

Dieting for dogs can be dangerous, just as it can be for people. You should consult your veterinarian before taking any step that may cause your dog to lose weight.

Food Supplements

There are several types of supplements that are helpful to your dog's health. However, not all are beneficial. It is important to stick to the recommended dosage; oversupplementing can be harmful. Discuss supplementation with your veterinarian.

- Vitamins—Puppies and older dogs often need more nutrients than an adult dog. Vitamins designed specifically for dogs can meet this need. Also, they often taste good and can be used for treats.

- Oils—Certain oils can be added to the regular food. Oils help make the coat healthy and shiny. And they can make food taste better. There are several products available through veterinarians and pet stores that make good oil supplements. Small amounts of corn oil and olive oil (1 to 3 teaspoons depending on the size of the dog) also are good.

- Bones—Discussed in Chapter 1, Preventive Medicine (see page 13).

- Rawhide—Discussed in Chapter 1, Preventive Medicine (see page 14).

- Biscuits—Discussed in Chapter 1, Preventive Medicine (see page 14).

Tablescraps

Tablescraps are not good for a dog. They often upset the stomach, causing vomiting and diarrhea. In addition, they are the leading cause of obesity and foster annoying behavior, such as begging.

Summary

- Always have clean, fresh water available.
- Choose a commercial dog food that provides a complete, balanced diet.
- Do not vary or change food often.
- Adjust the amount of food given to suit your dog's needs.
- Adjust the number of times of feeding a day to suit your dog's needs.
- Regularly check your dog's weight.
- Supplement diet as recommended by your veterinarian.
- Do not feed your dog tablescraps.

3   Parasites

Introduction

A parasite is an organism that lives off of another
organism to the detriment of the host. A number of
parasites affect dogs. Besides being debilitating to
animals, some can affect people. As soon as a dog is
detected to have parasites, it should be treated
promptly and thoroughly.

Heartworms

Heartworms are one of the most dangerous parasites. In the immature microscopic stage, they are
carried by mosquitos and can be injected directly
into the bloodstream of a dog. They then travel to
the heart. Once in the heart, they grow to maturity
(6 to 8 inches long). As worms accumulate, they
begin to clog the heart and restrict the flow of blood.
The end result is heart failure and death. They can
infect people as well, although this is rare.

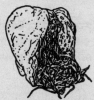

Heart clogged by heartworms.

A dog with heartworms can be treated. But this
often causes complications and can lead to death.
The best way to handle the problem is to prevent it.

Since heartworms are transmitted by mosquitos, a prevention program should extend from just before to just after mosquito season. If you live in an area where mosquitos are prevalent throughout the year, heartworm prevention should be a year-round program.

A prevention program begins with a blood test to confirm that your dog does not have heartworms. (Dogs in areas where mosquitos are a 12-month problem should have a blood test every 6 months.) Once this is confirmed, pills can be given that will kill the heartworms in the microscopic stage soon after these parasites are injected into the dog's bloodstream. In this manner, they are eradicated before they mature inside the heart. You will need to administer the pills either daily or monthly; the correct method for this is discussed in Chapter 22, Giving Medication (see page 151).

Worms

There are many types of worms. Some of the more common are discussed below.

- Roundworm—Looks like small spaghetti. Can cause vomiting, diarrhea, weight loss and lack of growth (in puppies).

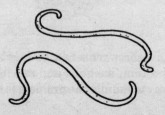

If dog is heavily infected, worms may be seen in vomit or stools. Transmitted through the ingestion of soiled material, feces or milk (from the mother when puppies are suckling). Can be transmitted to humans through ingestion of soiled material and feces.

- Tapeworm—Looks like rice grains attached to the anus. Can be fairly mobile and may move around like a slow motion slinky.

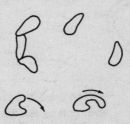

Usually does not show any clinical signs, but can cause diarrhea and weight loss in some cases. Transmitted through ingestion of an infected flea or through eating wild animals such as mice or rats. Can infect humans if an infected flea is swallowed; cannot be transmitted directly from the dog.

- Hookworm—Usually 1/2 to 1 inch in length and in the shape of a hook. Smaller than roundworms. Can cause vomiting, weight loss, emaciation, anemia, pnuemonia and diarrhea. Sometimes causes the production of dark, tarry feces. Transmitted by penetration through the skin or ingestion. Can also affect humans.

- Whipworm—Usually 2 to 3 inches long. Inhabit the small and large bowels. The eggs are resilient; they can remain viable for up to 5 years.

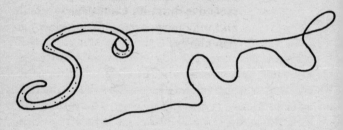

Often does not show any clinical signs but can cause diarrhea with blood and weight loss. Transmitted by ingestion of soiled material. Often contracted in areas where many dogs congregate.

There are several signs to look for if you think that your dog might have worms.

Signs of Worms

- Vomiting and/or diarrhea
- Pot belly abdomen (mainly in puppies)
- Loss of weight (even if eating more food

than normal)
- Spaghetti-like particles in vomit or feces
- Rice-like particles around the anus

What to Do

- Collect a fecal sample (also known as a stool sample).
- Take the sample and your dog to your veterinarian for an examination.

Your veterinarian will test the stool sample. If the tests are positive, your dog will be treated with an injection and/or oral medicine. Most successful treatment requires two stages. The first kills the existing worms but not their eggs. The second set kills the recently hatched worms before they can breed. The timing between the two is crucial; follow your veterinarian's instruction diligently.

The chance of contracting worms can be reduced.

Steps of Prevention

- Clean up after your dog.
- Insist that others clean up after their dogs. Most worms are transmitted by coming into contact with the feces of infected animals.
- Do not let your dog eat raw meat.
- Have your dog tested every 6 months.
- Treat for fleas as needed.

Other Intestinal Parasites

Besides worms, other parasites afflict the intestinal tract. Signs, treatment and prevention of these are similar to that of worms.

- Coccidia—Tiny parasite that can be seen only through a microscope. Can cause diarrhea (occasionally with blood), weight loss and dehydration. Transmitted by ingestion of fecal-contaminated material.

- Giardia—Also a microscopic parasite living in the intestines. Similar symptoms and characteristics to those of coccidia. Can be transmitted to people.

Ringworm

Contrary to its name, ringworm is not a worm; it is a fungus that causes skin disease. It is transmitted through contact with an infected animal or its environment. Common sites of ringworm are animal shelters and other locations where large groups of animals are kept. Puppies are most commonly affected; ringworm can readily affect people as well, particularly small children.

Signs of Ringworm

- Hair loss in patches
- Lesions around eyes, ears, head and feet
- Scaling and crusting of skin

- **Excessive scratching**

What to Do

- Transport to your veterinarian (see page 135).

Fleas

The most likely reason that a dog scratches itself is that it has fleas. Fleas are insects that are often seen running or jumping around an infected animal. They feed by biting the animal and sucking its blood.

Fleas are harmful in two ways. First, they often cause skin infections. Flea bites itch; heavy scratching irritates the skin and makes the dog prone to infections. Some dogs are allergic to flea bites. Thus, one bite alone can lead to a serious skin problem. Second, fleas feed on blood. When biting through the skin, they can transmit germs and diseases into the bloodstream. Both of these problems can affect people, too. A heavy flea infestation can cause anemia, which can be fatal (especially for puppies).

Fleas thrive in warm weather. As a result, they are a year-round problem in warm climates. While prevalent mainy during the summer months in cold climates, fleas can continue to live indoors if the temperature inside is constantly warm. They can infest even the cleanest home.

In order to control fleas, you must treat both the dog and the dog's environment. Fleas can move around quickly and easily. If you treat the dog but not your home and yard, the problem will persist. Also, if you have more than one animal, you should treat them all at the same time.

There are a number of good products available for controlling fleas. Your veterinarian can tell you which products work best in your area.

Steps to Control Fleas

- Use a flea and tick powder or spray designed for dogs once a week. It is important to read the label of any flea product that you use and to carefully follow the instructions; incorrect use can lead to poisoning. Small puppies may need special treatment; check with your veterinarian.
- Bathe dog periodically with a medicated shampoo. Follow instructions carefully.
- Use a flea and tick collar. This will limit the number of fleas but it may not totally control them. Check the neck once a week for any signs of skin reaction.
- Treat your home and yard with a top-

quality flea control product.
- Clean the dog's bedding once a week.

Ticks

Ticks are large parasites that feed by sucking blood. They bury their heads in the skin (usually around the head, neck and ears) and are difficult to remove. Since they penetrate the skin, they can transmit diseases such as Lymes Disease. Lymes is a bacterial disease that can cause fever, lethargy, heart problems, kidney failure, meningitis and sore joints. It can affect people as well, but it is usually transmitted directly from the Deer Tick.

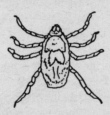

Tick season occurs in warm weather. During this time, you should examine your dog everytime it comes in from outside. If you see a tick, remove it at once.

Steps to Control Ticks

- Use a flea and tick collar.
- Spray once a week with a flea and tick product.
- Examine the dog when it comes in from outside.

What to Do—Removing a Tick

- Spray a heavy dose of tick spray directly on the tick or cover it with strong alcohol. Be careful not to get any spray or alcohol into your dog's mouth, nose, eyes or ear canal.
- Wait 5 minutes.
- Pull tick off using a pair of tweezers. (Do not use your fingers; direct contact with a tick may increase the chance of you contracting a disease from it.)
  - Grasp tick as close to the skin as possible.

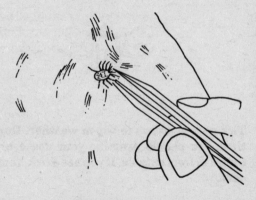

  - Pull using steady, even pressure. Do not use a sudden jerk or twist.
- Contact your veterinarian if you have any problems. The most common problem is leaving the head of the tick in the skin; this often leads to infection.

Ear Mites

Ear mites are tiny insects that affect dogs in two ways. First, they cause itching which, when alleviated by heavy scratching, can lead to ruptured blood vessels. Second, the mites cause the ear to secrete a thick waxy discharge that often clogs the ear canal. Both can lead to ear infection. Mites are transmitted by direct contact with infected animals; this oftens occurs among puppies that are still in the litter and animals that are in large groups.

Steps to Control Ear Mites

- Have dog or puppy examined by your veterinarian soon after acquisition.
- Have the ears examined if there is persistent scratching.
- Follow the directions for treatment given by your veterinarian. The proper way to administer ear medication is shown in Chapter 22, Giving Medication (see page 151).

Mange

The many varieties of mange are caused by mites that burrow into the skin or that live in the hair or on the scalp. They are most often found around the head, neck, eyes, ears or feet. They can cause a tremendous amount of scratching, making the dog susceptible to infection. Some forms of mange can be transmitted to people.

Signs of Mange

- Heavy scratching
- Loss of hair
- Dry, scaly skin over parts of the body
- Sores covering parts of the body

What to Do

- Transport to your veterinarian (see page 135).

Summary

- It is not uncommon for a dog to have parasites.
- Parasites can pose health hazards to people.
- All parasites should be eradicated as soon as detected.
- A heartworm prevention program is critical to your dog's health.
- Your dog should be checked for worms regularly.
- When controlling fleas, you must treat both the dog and its environment.
- Successful flea treatment must be consistent and thorough.
- After removing a tick, contact your veterinarian if you have left the head of the tick in the dog.
- Have your dog examined if there is persistent scratching.

4   The Older Dog

Introduction

As a dog ages, its body begins to lose its ability to fight off disease and to repair itself. An older dog can have an enjoyable and rewarding life but this stage of life requires some adjustments. While this chapter gives you some ideas, your veterinarian is the best source of information and advice.

Aging

Every dog ages at a different rate. Some giant dogs may show signs of aging at about 6 to 7 years; smaller dogs may not until around 12 years. The average is around 7 to 9 years.

Signs of an Older Dog

- Less active than usual
- Changes in normal habits, such as sleeping more
- Moves more slowly
- Changes in personality
- More sensitive to extreme heat and cold

These are normal signs of aging and should not alarm you (unless there is a sudden change). But you should discuss them with your veterinarian on your next visit.

The immune system of an older dog is less effective, making it more susceptible to disease and illness. In addition, the body organs do not function as well in an older dog as they do in a younger one. Some dogs begin to have problems with their kidneys, heart, liver or urinary tract. If any of the normal signs of aging appear with any of the signs of problems listed below, your dog should be examined by your veterinarian.

Signs of Problems in an Older Dog

- Loss of weight
- Vomiting and diarrhea
- Loss of appetite
- Increased drinking and urinating
- Pain
- Difficulty standing
- Difficulty breathing
- Bumping into objects
- Blood in urine
- Coughing
- Drooling
- Reduced sense of hearing

Loss of weight is a common sign in a dog that is slowly developing a disease. It is a good idea to weigh your dog once a week as it gets older. This will allow you to monitor any gradual changes.

Nutrition

The nutritional needs of an older dog are different from that of one in the prime of life. As a dog loses some of its energy, its need for food reduces and its ability to digest food may be impaired. Without a change in its diet, your dog may become overweight. Obesity compounds problems related to aging.

Changing the type of food may be a good idea. Several foods geared for the needs of an older dog are available. In addition, there are foods designed for dogs with specific problems like heart disease and kidney disease. Adding a vitamin supplement designed for dogs may also be beneficial.

Above all, you should provide enough clean, fresh water. Many older dogs suffer from kidney problems or failure. The result is that more water than normal is released into the urine. Additional water is needed to replace the large amount voided by urinating. Low levels of water may lead to dehydration. This can damage many internal organs, cause a build up of toxic by-products and potentially develop into a life threatening condition.

Check with your veterinarian before making any changes in your dog's diet or adding a supplement. Your doctor has your dog's medical background and can help you make the best decisions.

Exercise

Besides slowing down in general, older dogs often develop arthritis. This is the inflammation of joints that make movement difficult and painful. But all older dogs, even arthritic ones, need exercise.

It is a good idea to adjust your exercise program to be gentle and consistent. Walking is gentle; running is hard on the joints. One of the best exercises is swimming. It works the muscles without putting a great deal of stress on the joints. Avoid working the dog hard one day and resting it the next. A consistent amount of gentle exercise every day is more beneficial.

The Geriatric Work-Up

In older dogs, many major problems and diseases develop slowly. Early diagnosis greatly increases the chance of successful treatment and management of problems. To help catch them early, many veterinarians are now offering a geriatric work-up.

The geriatric work-up is a series of tests and exams that may show that a problem is developing. With the results, your veterinarian can advise you on what steps to take that will maximize your dog's good health and life expectancy. It can become a regular component of your annual visit.

The following is an example of a very thorough work-up illustrating the possibilities of modern veterinary medicine. The actual work-up chosen for your dog can vary tremendously depending on the result of the physical examination and your dog's medical history.

An Example of a Geriatric Work-Up

• Complete physical examination

- X-ray of chest
- X-ray of the abdomen
- X-ray of the hips
- Complete blood test
- Urine test
- Electrocardiogram

Summary

- Older dogs can enjoy life and be happy.
- Signs of aging usually are not serious unless there are other signs of problems.
- Loss of weight is a good clue to something being wrong.
- Access to clean, fresh water is essential to good health.
- Changing your dog's diet might be a good idea.
- Do not switch to a special food or supplement for older dogs before checking with your veterinarian.
- Older dogs need gentle exercise.
- A geriatric work-up once a year may help head off problems.

PART II

FIRST AID

5   Essential Procedures

Overview

There are several basic procedures that you should
know. These will allow you to monitor your dog's
health between visits to your veterinarian.

Weighing Your Dog

Obesity is a common problem among dogs. Regular
weighing will help you control your dog's weight.

What to Do

- Weigh the dog and yourself on a bathroom
  scale.
- Set the dog down.
- Weigh yourself alone.
- Subtract your weight from that of the dog
  and you combined. The difference is the
  weight of the dog.

Taking a Temperature

Normal temperature is 101 to 102.5 degrees Fahr-
enheit. Use a rectal thermometer.

What to Do

- Shake thermometer down to about 95 or
  96 degrees.
- Lubricate the themometer with petro-

leum jelly.
- Have somebody hold the dog.
- Raise and hold the tail.
- Insert into the anus. Use a gentle twisting motion. Insert about half of the thermometer.

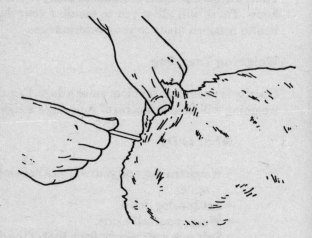

- Keep hold of both the thermometer and the tail.
- Leave in for 30 seconds to 1 minute.
- Pull out, wipe clean and read.

What NOT To Do

- Do NOT let go of the thermometer while it is inserted in your dog.
- Do NOT attempt to take a temperature if your dog struggles.
- Do NOT take temperature orally.

Taking a Pulse

A normal pulse is 70-160 heartbeats per minute; a puppy's may be as high as 220. There are two easy ways to take a pulse.

What to Do

Hand On Chest

- Grasp the chest just behind the elbows with one hand.
- Move hand until you feel the heart beat.

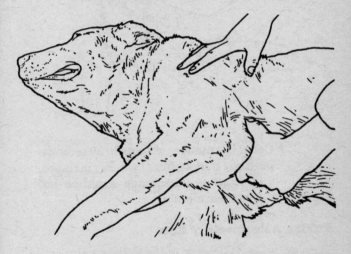

- Count the number of beats in 20 seconds.
- Multiply that number by 3. For instance, 40 beats in 20 seconds would be 120 beats per minute.

Hand On the Femoral Artery

- Place fingers on inside of back leg where it joins the body.
- Move fingers around until you find the artery.

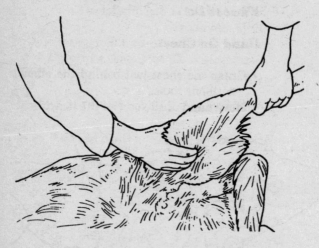

- Count the number of beats in 20 seconds.
- Multiply that number by 3. For instance, 50 beats in 20 seconds would be 150 beats per minute.

Taking a Respiratory Rate

The normal respiratory rate is between 10 and 30 breaths per minute. This rate can be much higher during and after exercising or playing. The number of breaths per minute can be measured by watching the chest or by placing a tissue in front of the nose.

What to Do

Watch the Chest

- Watch how many times the dog breathes in 20 seconds. (Count only the number of times that the dog inhales or exhales fully, not both.)
- Multiply that number by 3. For instance, 8 breathes in 20 seconds is a rate of 24 per minute.

Using a Tissue

- Hold a tissue in front of the nose.

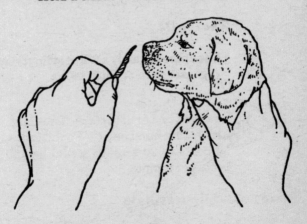

- Count how many times it moves in 20 seconds.
- Multiply that number by 3. For instance, if the tissue moves 6 times in 20 seconds, the rate is 18 per minute.

Muzzling Your Dog

Many dogs try to bite the veterinarian when being examined. This can be due to fear or anger. Regardless of the motive, a dog that bites is an animal to be wary of. In addition, many dogs in pain will try to bite when being moved or manipulated. You should take steps to protect both your veterinarian and yourself. Muzzling is a safe way to prevent biting.

There are many good commercial muzzles available through veterinarians or pet stores. It is recommended that you buy and keep it handy for extreme situations. However, if one is not available, you can improvise.

What to Do

- Use approximately a 2-foot strip of strong gauze, cloth or thick twine.

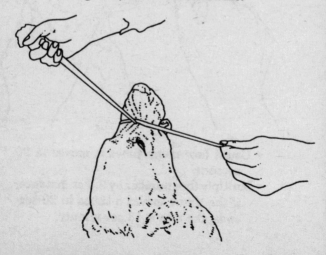

- Loop over nose by tying a half hitch knot. Both ends and the knot should be under the jaw.

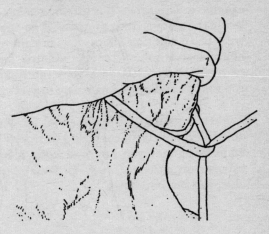

- Pull the ends around the neck.
- Tie in a bow behind the ears.

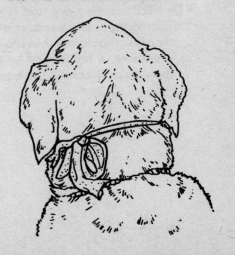

- Muzzle should be just tight enough to prevent the mouth from opening.

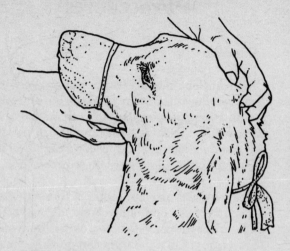

What NOT to Do

- Do NOT muzzle a dog that is vomiting, convulsing or unconscious; in addition, do NOT muzzle one that has difficulty breathing, a broken jaw or extensive damage in or around the mouth.

6   CPR: Life Saving Procedures

Overview

CPR (cardiopulmonary resuscitation) consists of two procedures that may save the life of your dog: mouth-to-nose respiration and heart massage. While they may be life-saving, they can also be detrimental; you may aggravate your dog's condition if you do not properly administer these procedures.

You should not attempt either of these unless you encounter two conditions. First, do not attempt CPR unless proper veterinary care is unavailable. If you can get to a veterinarian quickly, your dog will have a better chance of survival than if you try CPR yourself. Second, do not attempt either procedure unless it is obvious that your dog will die if you do nothing. In a horrible situation such as that, doing something is better than nothing at all.

If you attempt CPR and do not successfully revive your dog, do not think that you have failed. Trained professionals, using state-of-the-art techniques and drugs, often cannot save the dog. You can only do your best.

Mouth-To-Nose Respiration

After a serious accident, your dog may stop breathing. If you cannot detect any respiratory signs and proper veterinary care is too far away, you should try to get the lungs started again by giving mouth-to-nose respiration.

What to Do

- Clear the airway.
  - Pull the tongue forward in the mouth.

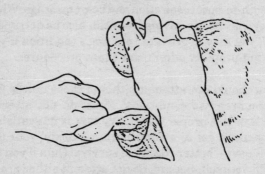

  - Remove any material that may be blocking the throat.
- Close mouth firmly.

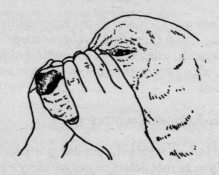

- Place your mouth over the nose of the dog.
- Blow into nose until the chest expands fully (usually 1 to 3 seconds).

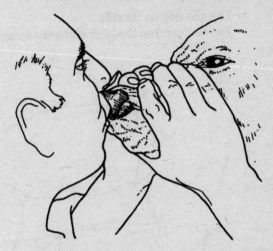

- Take mouth from nose, allowing the dog to exhale.
- Repeat the procedure for 10 seconds.
- Check dog for breathing on its own. If not, repeat (several times if necessary).
- Transport to your veterinarian immediately (see page 135).

Heart Massage

After a serious accident, the heart may stop beating. If there is no pulse and proper veterinary care is too far away, you should attempt to massage the heart.

What to Do

Small Dog or Dog with Narrow Chest

- Lay the dog on its side.
- Put one hand on the back along the spine.

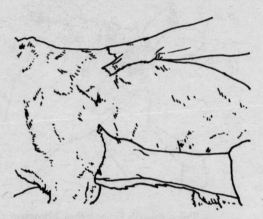

- Grasp the chest with the other hand.
- Push in firmly but gently. (Too much force may break the ribs.)
- Repeat rapidly for 15 seconds.
- Check for pulse.
- Repeat, if necessary.
- Transport to your veterinarian immediately (see page 135).

Large Dog

- Lay the dog on its back.
- Place heel of hand on the low end of the breastbone.

• Put other hand on top of first hand.

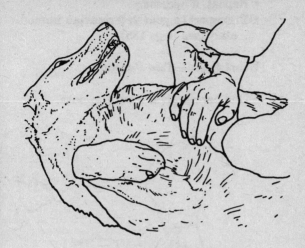

• Push down firmly but gently. (Too much force may break the ribs.)
• Repeat rapidly for 15 seconds.
• Check for pulse.
• Repeat, if necessary.
• Transport to your veterinarian immediately (see page 135).

CPR (Cardiopulmonary Resuscitation)

CPR is the combination of giving mouth-to-nose respiration and massaging the heart.

What to Do—One Person

• Do mouth-to-nose for 10 seconds.
• Massage heart for 15 seconds.

- Check for breathing and a pulse rate.
- Repeat, if necessary.
- Transport to your veterinarian immediately (see page 135).

What to Do—Two Persons

- One person gives mouth-to-nose.

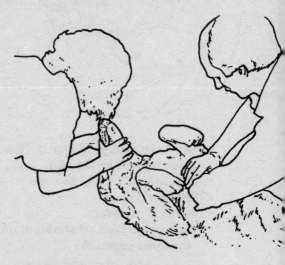

- The other massages the heart.
- Continue for 10-15 seconds.
- Check for breathing and a pulse rate.
- Repeat, if necessary.
- Transport to your veterinarian immediately (see page 135).

Crucial Point to Remember

Do NOT attempt mouth-to-nose, heart massage or CPR unless.....

- Proper veterinary care is not avaliable.
- It is obvious that your dog will not survive if you do nothing.

7 Unidentified Emergency

Overview

It is possible that you might encounter an emergency situation in which you have no idea as to what might be wrong or what caused the problem. In an instance such as this, you should transport the dog to your veterinarian as quickly as possible. The doctor will probably ask you numerous questions while examining your pet. You should try to provide as much information as possible.

Signs of Unidentified Emergency

- Dog collapsed or prostrate
- Unattributed unusual behavior

What to Do

- Transport to your veterinarian (see page 135). While en route to the clinic, think back over the recent past. By reviewing your dog system by system, you might pick up some clues.

  #### General
  - Less alert than normal?
  - Less active than normal?
  - Change in appetite or drinking pattern?
  - Outside for unusual period of time?

- Access to any substance that may be poisonous, such as insecticides, medicines, antifreeze or mouse/rat poison?
- How long has there been a problem?

Respiratory
- Difficulty breathing?
- Coughing or wheezing?
- Discharge from nose?
- Rapid respiratory rate?

Gastrointestinal
- Vomiting or diarrhea?
- Change in diet?
- Eating things that it should not?
- Bleeding from mouth or gums?
- Broken teeth?

Cardiovascular
- Reduced tolerance to exercise?
- Change in color of gums?

Urogenital
- Straining to urinate?
- Urinating more frequently?
- Discharge from vulva or penis?

Neurological
- Change in behavior?
- Bumping into objects?
- Staring into space?
- Unstable posture or falling over?

Musculoskeletal
- Limping or lameness?
- Pain in touched in certain areas?
- Difficulty in climbing stairs?
- Difficulty in standing up after lying for a period of time?

Integumentary
- Cuts or bruises?
- Bleeding?
- Hair loss?
- Excessive scratching?
- Biting at certain areas?
- Dull coat?
- Dirt or unusual substance on coat?

Ocular
- Sensitivity to light?
- Discharge from eyes?
- Third eyelid across?

What NOT to Do

- Do NOT waste time in attempting to diagnose your dog's condition. An unidentified emergency is often very serious. The key to survival may be reaching proper medical evaluation and treatment as fast as possible.

8　Hit by Car & Trauma

Overview

The most common cause of major trauma for a dog is being hit by a car. This often results in very serious injuries such as a crushed chest, broken bones, brain concussions, open and closed wounds, internal bleeding and internal organ damage. In addition, the dog usually goes into shock, in which case the blood flow to the skin and many organs is shut down.

Use caution when handling an injured dog. A dog in pain may resist any manipulation and may bite you. If you are bitten by a dog, you should seek medical attention.

You may not see your dog get hit by a car. But you may suspect it if you notice several signs.

Signs of Hit by Car and Trauma

- Difficulty breathing
- Scrapes and cuts
- Pain
- Limping or dragging a leg
- Cannot stand up properly
- Bleeding from nose
- Broken teeth
- Broken jaw
- Bruises

What to Do—ABCs

A good sequence of steps for first aid is
known as the ABCs.

> A—Airway
> B—Breathing
> C—Circulation

**If your dog shows no signs of life, transport to
your veterinarian immediately (see page 135).
If proper medical care is unavailable, attempt
CPR (see page 59).**

Airway

Airway first aid is clearing the airway tract so that
the dog can breathe.

What to Do

- Pull tongue out.

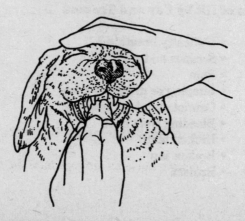

- Remove any blood or damaged tissue from the back of the mouth.

Breathing

Breathing first aid is ensuring that the dog is breathing properly.

If breathing OK, go to steps for Circulation (see page 76).

If there is a wound penetrating the chest cavity, air can enter the chest around the lungs. This makes normal breathing difficult or impossible. You should try to make an airtight seal over the wound.

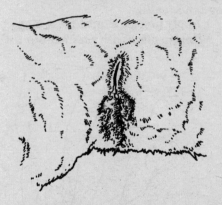

Sign of Air Entering an Open Wound

- Sucking noise as air goes in and out

What to Do

- Place a piece of cloth or plastic over the wound.

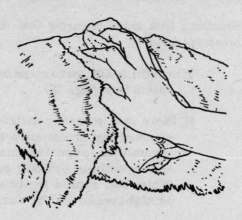

- Apply pressure until noise stops.
- Hold in place with your hand or with tape.

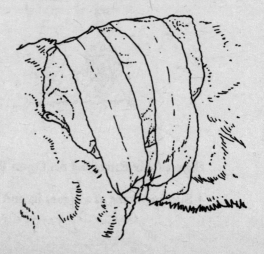

- Do NOT hold or tape too tightly. This makes breathing too difficult.
- Do NOT pull out objects from a chest wound.

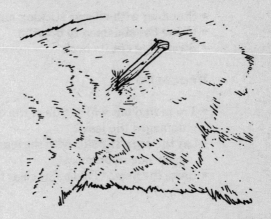

This may cause more damage. Place a bandage or a piece of plastic around any object sticking out of the chest.

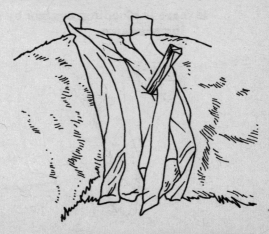

If the chest has been crushed, the dog will have difficulty breathing.

Signs of Crushed Chest

- Standing with elbows sticking out
- Using the abdomen to breathe
- Stretching out its neck

What to Do

- Try to find out which side of the chest is damaged the least.
- Lay the dog on its side with the least damaged side uppermost.
- Raise the head. (This helps clear the airway.)

Circulation

Circulation first aid is controlling any bleeding.

If there is bleeding, control by applying pressure.

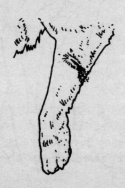

What to Do

- Wad up some cloth or gauze.
- Place directly on the wound.

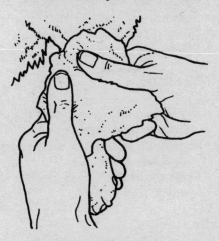

- Hold firmly but gently.

After ABCs

What to Do

- Transport to your veterinarian (see page 135).

What NOT to Do

- Do NOT assume that your dog is out of danger if it appears to be in good shape. It may have suffered internal damage. The extent of the injury may not be apparent for several hours or even days. By then, your dog may be in critical condition.

9 Broken Legs, Sprains, Strains & Dislocations

Overview

Most broken bones (fractures) are caused by being hit by a car or by falling. Fractures can be divided into two main groups: open and closed. An open fracture is when a bone breaks and cuts through the skin; it can easily be infected. If the skin is not pierced, it is a closed fracture. A major goal of closed fracture first aid is to keep it from becoming an open fracture.

A sprain is where muscles or ligaments twist beyond normal limits. A strain is the excessive stretching of muscles and tendons. A bone popping out of a joint or socket is a dislocation. It is difficult to tell the difference between a closed fracture and a sprain, strain or dislocation. Thus, they should be handled in a similar manner until veterinary care is reached.

Use caution when handling an injured animal. A dog in pain may resist any manipulation and can inflict considerable damage. If you are bitten by a dog, seek medical attention.

Signs of Breaks, Sprains, Strains & Dislocations

- Cracking or breaking sound at moment of

impact
- Change in size, shape or length of leg; may rest at a strange angle
- Broken bone may be visible

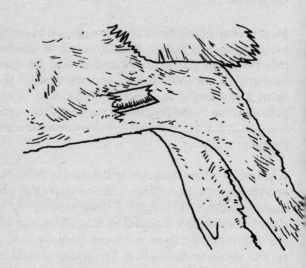

- Limping
- Standing on only three legs; the injured leg hanging limp
- Swelling around the injured area
- Pain

What to Do

- Muzzle the dog, if necessary (see page 56).
- Move the injured leg as little as possible.

- Place a folded towel or blanket under the leg for support.

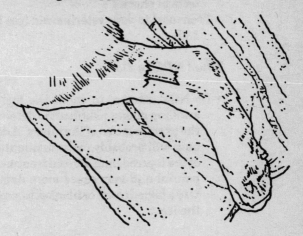

- If the bone is exposed, cover it with a light gauze or bandage.

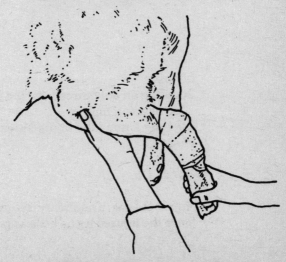

- Keep the dog as warm as possible; cover it with a blanket. (This reduces the effects of shock.)
- Transport to your veterinarian (see page 135).

What NOT to Do

- Do NOT attempt to splint the leg. The swelling makes it difficult to determine the exact location of the injury. A dog in pain will probably resist manipulation of the injured limb. Forced treatment is painful and may cause more damage. Use a folded towel or blanket to support the leg.

10 Wounds

Overview

A wound is a break in the continuity of tissue in any part of the body. Frequently, it is painful. You must exercise caution when handling a wounded animal. A dog in pain may bite. If you are bitten, you should seek medical attention.

There are two basic types of wounds: closed and open. With most wounds, there is a danger of infection. In addition, special steps should be taken if the wound is the result of a snake bite or an insect sting.

Closed Wounds

A closed wound can be an abrasion or contusion (also known as a bruise); it is a wound where the skin remains unbroken. However, there may be significant internal damage that goes undetected. The injured skin may die and fall off a few days after the injury occurred; it may also become infected. The area affected is not always obvious and the full extent of the damage may not be apparent for several days. A common cause of a closed wound is heavy friction on the skin or a blow from a blunt object.

Signs of a Closed Wound

- Pain

- **Heat in a small area**
- **Skin scratched up**
- **Swelling**

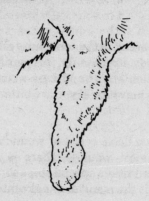

What to Do

- Bathe the area in cold water.
- Apply an ice pack. Use an icebag or place ice in a towel.

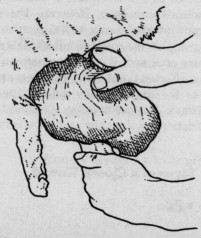

- If skin is scratched up, clean with 3% hydrogen peroxide or salt water (1 teaspoon salt to 1 pint warm water).
- Transport to your veterinarian (see page 135). If the wound appears serious, go to your doctor immediately. If not, go as soon as possible. All minor wounds should be checked by a veterinarian within 24 hours.

What NOT to Do

- Do NOT underestimate a closed wound. While it may look harmless, it can hide major internal damage. The full extent of the damage may not be apparent for several days. By then, your dog's condition may be very serious.

Open Wounds

An open wound is where the skin is broken, usually accompanied by significant bleeding. The loss of large amounts of blood can be life threatening. In addition, muscles, tendons, blood vessels and nerves may be severed and internal organs may be damaged. Since the outer layer of the body is open, dirt and bacteria can enter, leading to possible infection.

Signs of an Open Wound

- Bleeding
- Pain

- Limping
- Excessive licking of certain areas

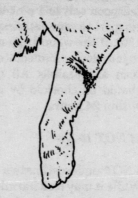

What to Do

- Use pressure to control the bleeding.
    - Wad up a clean cloth or some gauze.

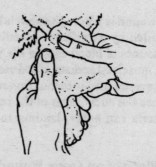

- Place directly on the wound.
- Hold firmly but gently until bleeding stops.

- If the wound is minor, clean the wound.
  - Flush the wound with 3% hydrogen peroxide or salt water (1 teaspoon salt to 1 pint warm water).

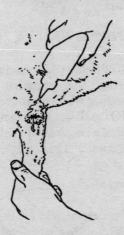

- Dab clean with gauze or cloth. (Do NOT rub. This hurts and may cause more damage.)

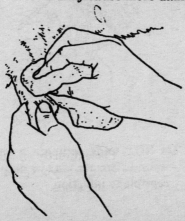

- Transport to your veterinarian (see page 135). A dog with a major wound should go to the doctor immediately. A minor wound should be checked within 24 hours.

What NOT to Do

- Do NOT delay transporting to the veterinarian. Use pressure to control the bleeding while en route.
- Do NOT pull out an object that has penetrated a body cavity such as the chest or abdomen. This might cause more damage.

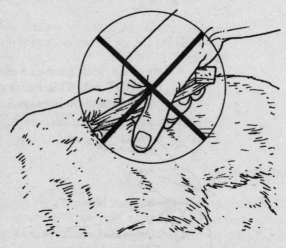

- Do NOT underestimate a small open wound. The cut may be deep and susceptible to infection.

Infection

Infection can be a complication of any wound. It involves the growth of bacteria that leads to heat, redness, swelling and pain. An infected limb can be so swollen and painful that it may resemble a broken leg. Infection can spread into the bloodstream, occasionally causing the dog to run a fever and to go off its food. A very serious infection can end in major surgery or possibly death.

Signs of Infection

- Swelling
- Limping
- Pain
- Colored discharge (usually cream, yellow, green, brown or blood-tinged)
- Foul odor

What To Do

- Transport to your veterinarian (see page 135).

Snake Bite

Most snakes are not poisonous. However, pit vipers (rattlesnakes, copperheads, and water moccasins) are. A pit viper has two fangs that puncture the skin and pump the venom. Coral snakes are also poisonous.

The parts of a dog usually bitten are the head and

the legs. If you cannot identify the snake when the dog is bitten and the wound consists of two small openings close together, assume that the snake is poisonous.

A dog bitten by a poisonous snake is in a very serious predicament. The two keys to survival are keeping the dog quiet and obtaining prompt medical attention.

Signs of a Snake Bite

- Two deep punctures

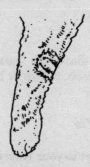

- Swelling
- Area tender and painful to touch
- Weakness
- Wobbling
- Acting nervous

What to Do

- Identify the type of snake, if possible.
- Keep animal quiet.

- Restrict its movement. (This reduces the amount of venom pumped around the body.)
- Apply a tourniquet only if bite is on the lower part of a leg and you think that the snake was poisonous.
    - Wrap a thin belt, bandage or string several times around the leg above the wound.

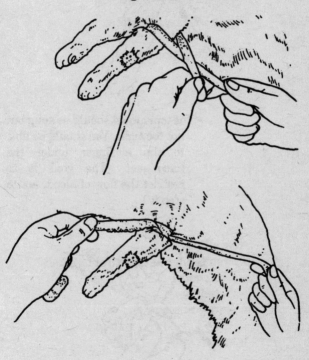

- **Tie into a bow.**

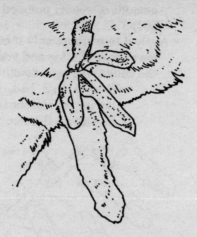

- The tourniquet should be snug but not too tight. You should be able to slip a finger under the tourniquet. (The goal is to restrict the flow of blood, not to stop it.)

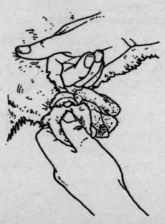

- Keep the dog warm. This reduces the effect of shock.
- Transport to your veterinarian (see page 135). If you cannot reach medical attention within a short period of time, loosen the tourniquet for 30 seconds every 10 minutes.

What NOT to Do

- Do NOT cut the wound and try to suck out the snake venom. This rarely helps and may cause more damage.
- Do NOT apply a tourniquet if the dog resists. Exciting the dog will hasten the spread of the toxins around the body.

Insect Stings

Most insect stings are painful but harmless. However, it is possible that a dog may have an allergic reaction to the insect venom, causing its airway passages to contract. This makes breathing difficult and reduces the effectiveness of the cardiovascular system. The end result can be shock and sometimes death.

Signs of an Insect Sting

- Swelling, usually around the face or legs
- Heat felt when touched
- Possible shock within 30 minutes (if allergic reaction takes place)

What to Do

- Remove stinger, if still in dog.
  - Use tweezers.
    - Grasp stinger at the point of entry to the skin.

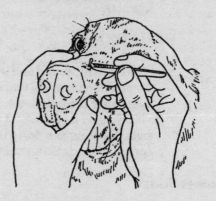

  - Pull straight out using a steady, even pressure.
- Apply a cold compress or cloth soaked in cold water.
- Transport to your veterinarian (see page 135).

What NOT to Do

- When removing a stinger, do NOT squeeze the venom sack. This will inject more venom into the dog.

11   Burns

Overview

A burn is the destruction of tissue by extreme and localized heat. The severity of a burn is measured by how deep the skin is affected and how much surface area is covered. Often the full extent of a burn is not known until several days after the accident.

There are three types of burns.

- Thermal Burns
- Chemical Burns
- Electrical Burns

A thermal burn is the most common. It is caused by being scalded by boiling water, touching an open flame or coming in contact with a hot surface such as an oven door, stovetop or a heating pad. Overexposure to a heating lamp is another frequent cause. A thermal burn will turn the skin red. It may blister and cause the hair around the burn to be singed.

A chemical burn is caused by the spillage of corrosive liquids on the dog. A substance containing an alkali such as lye or ammonia will turn the affected area white or brown. It will give the skin a soapy or slippery feel. An acidic substance will cause the skin to dehydrate, contract and darken. Acid burns are very painful, unless the nerve endings in the skin have been killed. This would result in no pain but is still very serious.

An electrical burn is discussed in Chapter 12, Electrocution (see page 99).

Signs of Burns

- Skin turning red, white or brown
- Hair singed or falling out in spots

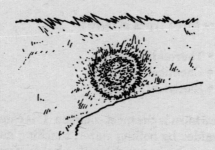

- Skin painful to touch
- Skin contracting
- Skin soapy or slippery to feel
- Blisters

What to Do

- Put on gloves, if available. If you do not wear gloves while treating a chemical burn, you may also be burned.
- Clean and treat burn.

For burns that leave the skin intact.

- Wash burned area with cold water. Use a gentle stream or place in a bath.

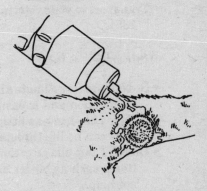

- Put a cold compress on the area burned. (The faster the skin is cooled down, the less damage will occur and the greater the chance for a favorable outcome.)

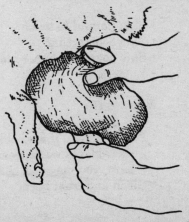

For burns that go through entire thickness of skin

- Cover with dry cloth or towel. (Washing the burn is usually too painful.)
- Transport to your veterinarian (see page 135).

What NOT To Do

- Do NOT underestimate a burn. It is prone to infection and is easily complicated. Burns covering as little as 15% of the body can be life threatening.
- Do NOT put oils or creams on the burn. Items such as butter or margarine do not help.

12   Electrocution

Overview

Electrocution occurs when an electrical current passes through the body. It commonly happens when a dog chews through an electrical cord. It can also be caused by being in contact with power lines, touching exposed wires and being struck by lightening.

There are two problems caused by electrocution. First, the electrical current can create tremendous heat and cause an electrical burn. Second, the current may result in the shut down of key organs such as the heart, the lungs and the kidneys.

The danger of electrocution is deceptive. An animal may appear to recover from a shock within a few minutes. However, the full effects may not appear until 24 to 48 hours after the event. Possible consequences are that the lungs gradually fill with fluid or the heart may develop an abnormal rhythm. Any dog that has been electrocuted should be examined by a veterinarian.

Electrocution Prevention

Since most electrocution occurs by chewing through electrical cords, puppies that are teething or going through a chewing phase are especially at risk. You can take a few steps to minimize the chance of an accident.

- Unplug cords and equipment not in use.
- Replace old or frayed wires.
- Use a product designed to deter chewing. This is applied directly to an object and has a bitter taste that most dogs do not like.

Signs of Electrocution

- Burns, usually around the mouth (most burns will have a pale center surrounded by redness and swelling)
- Convulsions
- Collapsed or lying on side
- Low respiratory rate (under 10 breaths per minute)
- Loss of consciousness
- Heart may have stopped
- Voiding urine and feces

What to Do

- Switch off electrical source.
- Check for vital signs. (Is the dog breathing and does it have a heartbeat?)
- Transport to your veterinarian (see page 135). If your dog does not have any vital signs and proper veterinary care is not available, attempt CPR (see page 59). Even if your dog appears to have fully recovered, you should take your dog to your clinic immediately.

What NOT to Do

- Do NOT touch the dog if it is still in contact with the electrical current. If you do, you may also be electrocuted. If the dog is touching the source of electricity and is very rigid, it is probably still being shocked. Also watch for any water that may be in contact with the dog.

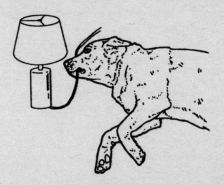

Before touching the dog, turn off the electricity by shutting it off at the source or pulling out the plug (do not touch any exposed wires). If you cannot shut off the electricity, move the dog with a non-metal object (such as a broomstick).

13   Heat Stroke

Overview

Dogs use the respiratory system to control body temperature. When hot, dogs inhale cool air through the nose and exhale hot air through the mouth. The faster dogs breathe, the quicker their bodies will cool down. This is why many dogs pant after exercising on hot days.

This process works well as long as the outside temperature is under the normal 101 to 102.5 degree body temperature of dogs. When the outside temperature approaches or exceeds this, a dog cannot efficiently cool itself down. The inability to lose excess body heat can result in heat stroke. This causes a reduction of blood circulation, reduced performance of the kidneys (the blood cleaning filter) and swelling of the brain. It is an extremely serious condition with a high mortality rate.

Heat stroke can affect all dogs, but some have a greater risk than others. These include long-haired breeds, all overweight dogs, older dogs, dogs with heart conditions and breeds that have flat, boxy noses (like Boxers, Pugs, Bulldogs, Boston Terriers and Pekingese).

The most common cause of heat stroke is leaving dogs in cars. On a hot day, the temperature in a car can reach 130 degrees in a short period of time. The temperature can soar even if the windows are open.

Another cause is confining a dog in a room without good ventilation or air conditioning during hot weather. Heavy exercising or playing on hot days and keeping a dog in a yard with no shade are also contributing factors.

Heat stroke can be prevented by using common sense. Do not leave your dog in the car on a hot day. Also do not keep it in a yard with no shade or in a room without good ventilation. You should leave a fan or air conditioner on low when confining your dog to the house. Its activities should be limited on extremely hot days. Above all, your dog should always have access to fresh water.

Signs of Heat Stroke

- Extreme panting
- Excessive salivation
- Collapse
- Anxious expression on face
- Rectal temperature of 105 degrees or higher

What to Do

- Get the dog's temperature down.

    - Immerse in or hose down with cold water. Keep dog in water until its temperature goes down. Hold the head above water.

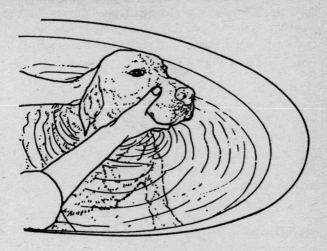

- Or give an alcohol bath.
  - Soak the legs with rubbing alcohol.

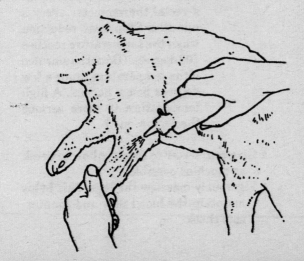

- Pour a small amount on the body.

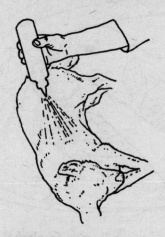

- Place an ice pack on the head and around the body.
- Check the body temperature with a rectal thermometer every 5 minutes. Stop heat reduction when the temperature reaches 103 degrees. (Do not be alarmed if the temperature drops a few degrees below normal. A high temperature is more serious than a low one.)

- Give cold water to drink. Allow to drink as much as possible.
- Vigorously massage the legs. This helps maintain the blood flow and counteracts shock.

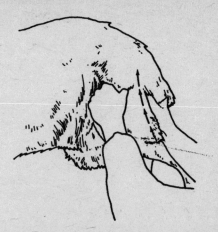

- Transport to your veterinarian (see page 135). The dog should be examined even if its temperature drops back to normal quickly.

What NOT to Do

- Do NOT put the its head under water when immersing the dog.
- Do NOT put alcohol on the dog's head when giving it an alcohol bath.

14   Cold Exposure & Frostbite

Overview

Cold exposure (also known as hypothermia) happens when the body temperature becomes much lower than the normal range of 101 to 102.5 degrees. The dogs most likely to be affected are those that lose body heat at fast rates. These include small breeds, short-haired breeds and all older dogs. Puppies are also at risk because of their large body surface relative to their body weight, which facilitates heat loss. Injured dogs are threatened as well. Exposure is very serious and frequently results in death.

In addition, exposure to cold may cause frostbite, a condition in which the skin tissue begins to die. It is possible to develop this condition without suffering serious hypothermia. The parts of a dog prone to frostbite are the tail, tips of the ears and footpads. Frostbitten tissue is very fragile and should be handled very carefully.

You can reduce the chance of your dog being overexposed or frostbitten by limiting its time outdoors in very cold weather. Also, small and short-haired dogs should wear sweaters or coats when being exercised.

Signs of Cold Exposure

- Stiff muscles
- Shivering
- Cold to touch
- Dilated and fixed eye pupils.
- Low pulse rate (below 70 beats per minute)
- Low respiratory rate (below 10 breaths per minute)
- Body temperature below 101 degrees

Signs of Frostbite

- Scaling of the skin
- Loss of hair
- White hair
- A leathery-feel to the skin

What to Do

- Handle carefully and very gently.
- Warm up slowly.

  - Wrap in a blanket.
  - A hot water bottle or a heating pad set on low can be used. Place it underneath the blanket, not directly on the dog.

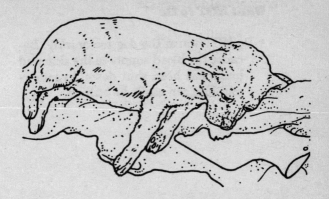

- A hair dryer can be used. Set on warm, not hot.

- Transport to your veterinarian (see page 135). If you cannot reach medical attention quickly, place the dog in a tub of warm water (105-110 degrees). Keep its head above water.

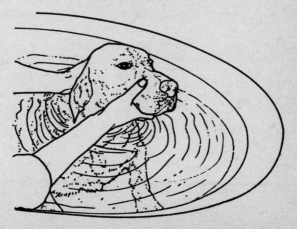

What NOT to Do

- Do NOT warm the dog too quickly. Because the blood supply to the skin and limbs has been shut down, hypothermic dogs can easily be burned.

15   Choking & Object in Mouth

Overview

Choking occurs when an animal cannot breathe normally due to an object in its throat blocking the airway. Puppies are especially at risk because they often try to swallow the objects that they chew on while teething. These objects can become stuck in the throat, causing the animal to choke. If your dog is choking, you must quickly attempt to dislodge the object blocking the airway. Do not wait for veterinary assistance. Choking can be fatal.

It is possible that an object can be stuck in the mouth without causing the animal to choke. Although the dog may be able to breathe, the object may shift and subsequently block the airway. Therefore, it is potentially dangerous and should be removed as quickly as possible.

Use care when handling an injured animal. A dog that is choking or has an object stuck in its mouth may panic and can inflict considerable damage. It may try to bite you when you attempt to remove the object. If you are bitten, seek medical attention.

Signs of Choking

- Not able to breathe
- Rubbing face on ground

- Pawing at mouth
- Eyes bulging
- Blue tongue
- Choking sound

What to Do

- Try to remove the object by hand.

  - Hold dog securely.
  - Open mouth wide.

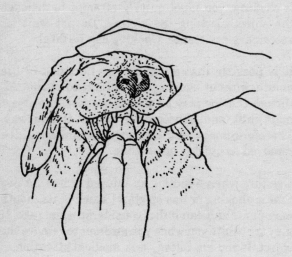

  - Grab object with hand.
  - Pull out gently.

- **(For small dogs only)** If unsuccessful, pick up by grasping the thighs just above the knees. Gently swing back and forth several times.

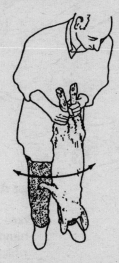

- If unsuccessful, use the Heimlich maneuver. (This forces air out of the lungs and blows the object out of the airway tract.)

    - Lay the dog on its side.
    - Position hands on dog.

    Small dog

    - Place one hand on the back.

- **Grasp the abdomen just below the ribs with the other.**

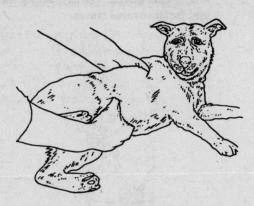

Large dog

- **Place the heel of both hands just below the ribs.**

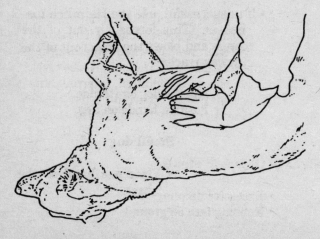

- Use hand(s) below ribs to sharply press in and upward (too much force may cause internal damage).
- If object is still stuck, repeat rapidly several times.
- Transport to your veterinarian (see page 135). If that is not possible and the dog has no pulse or respiratory signs, attempt CPR (see page 59).

What NOT to Do

- Do NOT wait for a veterinarian to remove the object blocking the airway. A choking dog cannot breathe and will probably die within a short period of time. You must take action.
- Do NOT swing a large dog by its hind legs. This may cause a dislocation of the hip or ligament damage
- Do NOT assume that the crisis is over when the object is removed. The throat will often swell up when something has been stuck in it. This might also block the airway. In addition, internal damage may have occurred by use of the Heimlich maneuver. The dog should be examined by your veterinarian.

Signs of Object in Mouth

- Excessive drooling
- Rubbing face on ground

- Pawing at mouth
- Difficulty in swallowing
- Interest in food but not eating

What to Do

- Try to remove the object by hand. Use the same procedure as with choking (see page 114).
- Transport to your veterinarian (see page 135).

What NOT to Do

- Do NOT force the removal of the object by hand. If it does not come out easily, leave it in place and transport to your veterinarian immediately.
- Do NOT pull out string or thread if part of it has been swallowed. It might saw through the stomach or intestines.
- Do NOT pull out fish hooks or any object embedded in tissue. This might cause more damage and serious bleeding.
- Do NOT struggle with your dog. If it is uncooperative, take it to your veterinarian.

16   Poison

Overview

A poison is any substance that can cause illness or death if it gets into the body. Most animal poisonings are self-inflicted by ingestion, inhalation, absorption or injection. Common ways include getting into poorly stored poisons around the house, eating a poisonous house plant and licking off excess flea and tick medicine from the skin.

There are thousands of poisonous substances. The large variety of symptoms make diagnosis difficult. Frequently, a veterinarian has to attempt treatment when it is not clear what the poison is or that the animal has been poisoned. It is important to convey as much information as possible to your doctor.

Generally, you will not see your dog poison itself. You might assume it if your dog is acting in a peculiar manner (especially if it has been missing for a period of time).

If you see your dog eat or come in contact with a poison, take it to your veterinarian immediately. Do not wait until signs of a problem develop.

Poison Prevention

Many cases of poisoning are caused by dogs eating something that is around the house. There are

several steps that can be taken to prevent this from
happening.

- Make a list of all plants in the home and
  garden.
  - Find out which are poisonous.
  - Remove them or keep them out of
    reach.
- Keep all chemicals, cleaning fluids, insecticides, fertilizers and medicines out of
  reach. Other common household poisons are antifreeze, mouse and rat
  poison, roach poison and slug poison.
- Do not overuse medical compounds such
  as flea and tick products. Closely follow
  the manufacturer's instructions.
- Do not let your dog roam the neighborhood. Unsupervised dogs often eat
  garbage and can easily ingest a poisonous substance.

Signs of Poisoning

- Severe vomiting
- Severe diarrhea
- Shaking
- Convulsions
- Blood in vomit, feces or urine
- Bluish color to tongue
- Weakness
- Collapse
- Difficulty breathing
- Excessive drooling

- Severe irritation of the eyes or mouth
- Peculiar substance on skin or coat

What to Do

- If the poison is on the skin, wash it off.
    - Use a lot of water.
    - Wear rubber gloves to avoid poisoning yourself.
- Allow dog to drink as much water as possible. (Water dilutes most poisons.)
- Give activated charcoal tablets, if available. (Charcoal absorbs many poisons.)
- Get a sample of the poison, if possible.
- Get a sample of vomit or stool, if poison not available.
- Transport to your veterinarian (see page 135). Telephone before departing. Your doctor may have special instructions, such as inducing vomiting to limit absorption.

What NOT to Do

- Do NOT wait for signs of poisoning to develop. Take your dog to your veterinarian if you see it ingest or come in contact with a toxic substance.
- Do NOT induce vomiting unless directed to do so by your veterinarian. Many poisons will burn the throat.
- Do NOT give anything by mouth if the dog is convulsing or unconscious.

- Do NOT give any human medication without checking with your veterinarian first.

17 Vomiting & Diarrhea

Overview

Vomiting and diarrhea clean out a dog's gastrointestinal system. The most common cause of vomiting and/or diarrhea is a sudden change of diet. A dog, accustomed to the effects of a particular food, may suffer an upset stomach if a different type of diet is abruptly introduced. Other causes include intestinal parasites, bacterial infections, motion sickness, internal foreign bodies, kidney failure and poisoning. Vomiting and diarrhea can range from not serious to very serious. Any vomiting or diarrhea by a puppy should be considered serious.

Prevention of Vomiting and Diarrhea

There are a few steps that you can take to eliminate many of the common causes.

- Do NOT feed your dog tablescraps.
- Avoid changing the type of food suddenly.
- Do NOT allow your dog to play with small objects that could be swallowed.
- Do NOT give rib or poultry bones.
- Do NOT let your dog roam around the neighborhood where it can get into garbage.
- Have your veterinarian perform regular fecal checks.

Signs—Not Serious

- Happens only once or twice
- No other signs of problems

What to Do

- Withhold all food for 24 hours.
- Give water.
- If symptoms stop after 24 hours, feed boiled white meat off the bone (chicken or turkey) with boiled white rice for 2 to 3 days. Gradually switch back to regular food.

Signs—Serious

- Symptoms lasting more than 24 hours
- Vomiting or has diarrhea frequently
- Blood in stool or vomit
- Fever
- Evidence of pain
- Weakness or collapse
- Dehydration (eyes sunk in sockets and skin not springing back into place when pinched)
- Signs of other problems (like runny eyes or nose and high respiratory rate)
- Any vomiting or diarrhea by a puppy

What to Do

- Transport to your veterinarian (see page 135).

18 Drowning

Overview

Drowning occurs when the lungs of an animal become flooded with fluid. This stops the inhalation of air and shuts down the respiratory system. Even if a drowning episode does not stop the animal from breathing, it can be serious. Excess fluid can damage the lungs, reducing their ability to absorb oxygen. As a result, a life threatening situation may exist several hours after the original incident occurred.

Drowning is uncommon among dogs because most are good swimmers over short distances. A common cause is a dog falling into a pool with steep steps that prevent it from escaping.

Signs of Drowning

- Panic and frantic effort to swim
- Motionless in water

What to Do

- Pull tongue out of mouth.

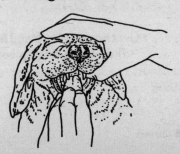

- Drain the water from the lungs.

Small Dog

- Pick up by grasping the hind legs around the thighs (just above the knee).

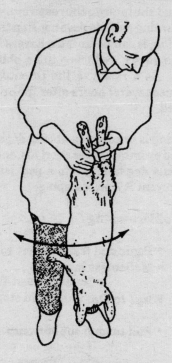

- Gently swing back and forth until fluid stops coming out.

Large Dog

- Pick up by its middle with head down.

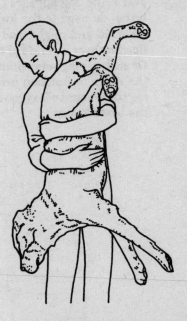

- Squeeze chest firmly but gently until fluid stops draining.

- Transport to your veterinarian (see page 135). If the dog has no pulse or respiratory rates and proper medical attention is not available, attempt CPR (see page 59).

What NOT to Do

- Do NOT assume that the emergency is over if the dog appears to recover. Internal damage to the lungs may have occurred and might lead to secondary flooding over a period of several hours. Or such damage may limit the ability of the lungs to function properly, reducing the amount of oxygen absorbed into the bloodstream.

19   Seizures

Overview

A seizure occurs when a dog appears to lose control of its body due to a malfunction of the brain. In controlling the nervous system, the brain acts like a computer. It stores a massive amount of information and sends messages to the various parts of the body via electrical impulses. When the brain malfunctions, the impulses that excite or turn on a body function may overwhelm those that suppress or turn off a function. This produces uncontrollable twitching and erratic behavior. The most common cause of seizures is epilepsy. However, seizures can be the result of several other afflictions such as tumors, meningitis or poisoning.

There are two types of seizures. A general seizure (or grand mal seizure) affects the entire brain. The second, partial seizure (also known as petit mal or focal seizure), only affects a portion of the brain. However, it can grow to be a general seizure.

For dogs that suffer recurring seizures, medication may be prescribed. These drugs do not always prevent seizures, but they help reduce the number and severity by stabilizing the cell membranes of the nerves in the brain. If your veterinarian does prescribe medication, you should give the medication regularly. Failure to do so may bring on a seizure.

If your dog has seizures, you should keep a log book. You should record when a seizure takes place and how long it lasts. If you notice that the seizures are occuring more frequently or for longer periods of time, contact your veterinarian within 24 hours.

Signs of a General Seizure

- Lying on side
- Cycling movement of legs
- Rolling of eyes
- Frothing of mouth
- Moving jaw rapidly
- Voiding urine and feces

Signs of a Partial Seizure

- Bumping into objects
- Standing and staring into space
- Trying to catch imaginary flies
- Localized twitching of muscles

What to Do

- Stop animal from hurting itself.

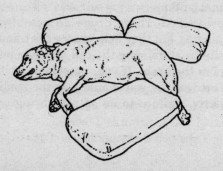

- Move it to a safe area, away from furniture and stairwells.
- Place blankets or pillows around it.
- Time the length of the seizure.

What NOT to Do

- Do NOT put your hand near the dog's mouth.

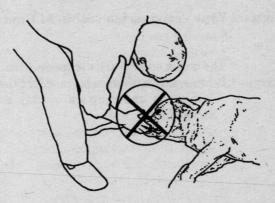

- Do NOT give anything by mouth.

After the Seizure

- Place dog in a dark room.
- Keep quiet. Do not make any sudden movements or loud noises.
- Give a moderate amount of food and water.
- Wipe away excess saliva.
- Clean up urine and feces.
- Take rectal temperature, if possible.

Contact Your Veterinarian Immediately If....

- It is your dog's first seizure.
- It has more than 1 seizure in a 24 hour period.
- The seizure lasts more than 3 minutes and the dog does not recover quickly and completely. Long, continual seizures can cause death.
- The temperature is over 103.5 degrees.

Contact Your Veterinarian within 24 Hours If....

- The dog is on anti-seizure medication.
- It has a single, short seizure of less than 3 minutes and recovers quickly and completely.

20   Twisted Stomach

Overview

Twisted stomach, also known as gastric tortion, is a condition in which the stomach becomes distended and turns around itself. The result is that the stomach's contents cannot empty into the small intestines. Gases and fluids build up in the stomach, causing rapid expansion. As the pressure grows, the dog will try to release it by belching and vomiting. The expanding stomach also presses on the diaphragm, restricting breathing. It can also inhibit the function of other internal organs such as the spleen and kidney.

A twisted stomach can obstruct the flow of blood to the stomach and lead to the death of tissue. As the stomach grows in size, pressure is applied to the venacava, the major vein that transports blood back to the heart. This leads to severe and catastrophic shock. With many dogs, this shock will be irreversible and result in death despite treatment.

Twisted stomach most often occurs among giant dogs and deep-chested breeds such as Great Danes, St. Bernards, German Shepards and Irish Setters. It can happen at any age.

This condition is an extreme emergency; professional help must be sought immediately.

Signs of Twisted Stomach

- Expanding abdomen
- Vomiting (or unsuccessfully trying to vomit)
- Frequent belching
- Rapid, shallow breathing
- Distressed look on face
- Shock
- Collapse

What to Do

- Transport to your veterinarian (see page 135).

21 Transporting to Your Veterinarian

Overview

Moving a critically injured animal can be dangerous; even slight motion can cause great damage. In addition, a dog in pain may try to bite you. It is crucial that you take precautions to reduce the chance of further injury and to protect both the animal and yourself. If you are bitten, you should seek medical attention.

Things To Remember

- **Support the back.** A seriously injured dog may have a broken back. If the back is not evenly supported when the dog is picked up, the broken bone may pull apart or the ends of the break may rub. This may cut the spinal cord, paralyzing the dog. The back can be supported by sliding a board or a folded thick towel beneath the dog prior to lifting. If that is not possible, try to keep the back straight when lifting the dog.

- **Keep a broken leg up.** If you suspect that the dog has a broken leg, place it on its side; the damaged limb should be up. This keeps the weight of the body off of the injured leg. You might give the limb some support by placing a folded towel or blanket underneath it.

- **Keep a crushed chest down.** If you suspect that the chest has been crushed, try to determine if one side of the chest is in better shape than the other. If this can be done, transport the dog with the least damaged side of the chest up. The lung on that side will function better than the one on the most damaged side. A dog lying with the most damaged side of the chest pointing up may have difficulty breathing. If there is both a broken leg and a crushed chest, the crushed chest should take priority.

- **Muzzle the dog, if necessary.** A dog in pain can be vicious, even to its owner. You may need to restrain it. However, do not muzzle a dog that is vomiting, convulsing or unconscious. Also do not muzzle a dog that may have a broken jaw or extensive damage inside the mouth. Muzzling is discussed on page 56.

Transporting a Dog With Minor Injuries

A dog with minor injuries will probably be able to walk to the car. If you choose to carry the dog, pick it up in your normal manner. Use special care not to aggravate the injury. Wrapping the dog in a blanket or towel can support an injured leg or help cover a wound. Also, it will keep the animal warm; reducing the effects of shock.

Transporting a Dog with Critical Injuries

Most small dogs can be transported by one person; large dogs may require more than one. It is a good idea to place a small dog in a box and a large dog on a board. Both methods will give the dog even support when picked up and will help keep the back straight. A blanket can provide support as well. However, do not waste time looking for one if it is not readily available. In a life threatening situation, reaching medical attention quickly is the key to the dog's survival.

What to Do

- Position dog to be picked up.

    - The back is toward you.
    - The side with a broken leg is up. (Place a towel or cloth under the leg for additional support.)
    - The side with a crushed chest is down.

- Slide dog onto a board. (Small dogs can be slid onto a folded towel or placed in a box.)

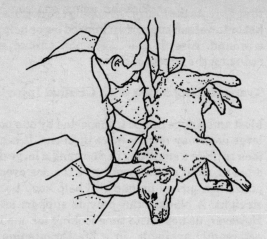

Small Dog

- Position hands beneath board or dog's body (if board not available.)

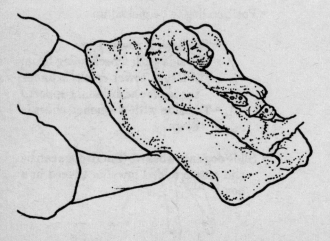

- **Pick up using one continuous, fluid motion.**

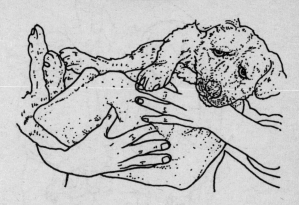

Large Dog

- **Position hands beneath board or dog's body (if board not available).**

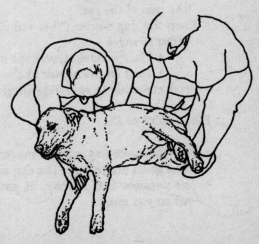

- Pick up using one continous, fluid motion.

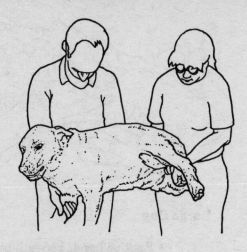

- Walk smoothly to car.
- Place the dog on seat with its back toward the rear of the car.
- Keep the dog warm. (This reduces the effect of shock.)
    - Place a blanket over the dog.
    - Turn on the heater in the car.
- Drive smoothly to your veterinarian.

What NOT to Do

- Do NOT make any sudden movements. The goals are to move the dog as little as possible and to move it smoothly when you must.

PART III

AFTER THE
EMERGENCY

22   Giving Medication

Overview

To complete the treatment of your dog, the veterinarian may prescribe medication and ask you to administer it. But the medication serves no purpose if you do not give it in the right dosage at the right times. Your veterinarian will instruct you on when and how to give medication.

Sometimes the prescribed drug will not have the desired effect. In cases such as this, your veterinarian may have to recommend another kind of drug or treatment. However, it is impossible to determine the effectiveness of a medication if the instructions are not followed.

Some dogs will not allow you to give them medication, despite your best efforts. Care must be taken to avoid being bitten by an uncooperative, angry animal. If you are bitten, you should seek medical attention.

If you are having difficulty giving medicine, contact your veterinarian. You might be advised to use an alternative method or to go to the clinic to have the medicine administered by injection.

Giving Pills

By Hand

- Position the dog so that it cannot back up. Place a large dog in a sitting position with its back to a wall. A small dog can be placed on a table next to a wall.
- Open the mouth.

  - Put one hand on the dog's muzzle. The thumb is just behind one canine tooth, the index finger behind the other.
  - Pull the head back.
  - The other hand pulls the jaw down.

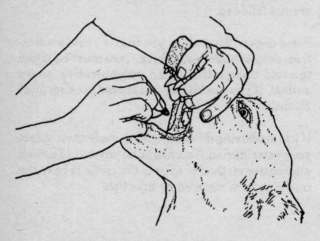

- Drop the pill as far back on the tongue as possible.

- **Touch the pill quickly and gently with the tip of your finger.**

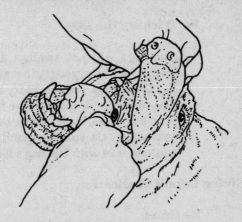

- **Close the mouth.**
- **Rub the throat until the dog swallows.**

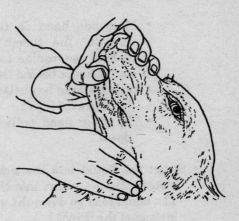

- Open mouth to check if the pill went down. If it did not, repeat.

By Tricking the Dog

- Some dogs will not swallow a pill no matter how hard you try to make them. For these dogs, you might try trickery. You can hide the pill in some food that your dog loves, such as cheese or peanut butter. Or you can grind the pill and mix it in with the dog's food.

Giving Liquid Medication

By Hand

- Open the mouth.

    - Place one hand on the dog's muzzle. The thumb is just behind one canine tooth, the index finger behind the other.
    - Keep the head level. (Do not tilt back like for pills.)
    - The other hand pulls the jaw down.

- Squirt the liquid into the side of the mouth. (Do not squirt into the back. The liquid may go down the windpipe instead of the throat.)

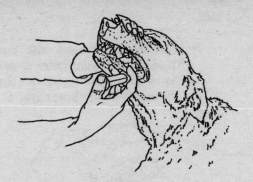

- Close the mouth.
- Rub the throat until the dog swallows.
- Open mouth to check if the liquid went down. If not, repeat.

By Tricking the Dog

- Fill a bowl with the dog's favorite food.
- Mix the liquid in thoroughly.

Medicating the Eyes

The common types of medication for the eyes are ointments and drops. It is important that these come into direct contact with the eyeball.

Ointment

- Clean away any discharge; use a tissue or cotton soaked in warm water.

- Separate the lower eyelid from the eye-ball.

   - Hold the dog's head with one hand so that your index finger is on the upper eyelid and the thumb is on the lower eyelid.

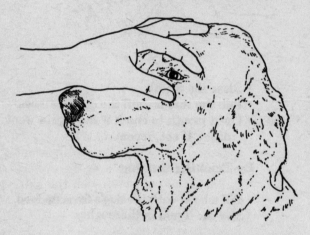

   - Move the thumb downward while holding the index finger steady. This creates a small cup between the lower eyelid and the eye.

- Rest the hand holding the tube of ointment on the side of the head.
- Run a bead of ointment in the cup. (Use care not to touch the eye with the tube; it might scratch the cornea.)

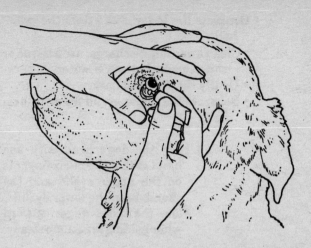

- Gently close the upper and lower eyelids together. This will cause the ointment to spread a thin film over the eyeball and socket. (Do not worry if the ointment turns white; the eye should clear within a few minutes.)

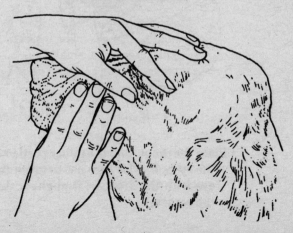

Drops

- Clean away any discharge; use a tissue or cotton soaked in warm water.
- Gently tilt the head back.
- Separate the upper eyelid from the eyeball.

  - Hold the dog's head with one hand so that the index finger is on the upper eyelid and the thumb is on the lower eyelid.
  - Move the index finger upward while holding the thumb steady.

- Rest the hand holding the eye dropper on the side of the head.

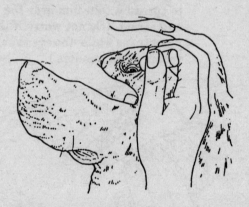

- Place the drops onto the upper portion of the eyeball. (Use care not to touch the eye with the dropper; it might scratch the cornea.)

Medicating the Ears

The ear canal of a dog has two sections (vertical and horizontal) with wax glands just in front of the eardrum. It is important that the medication traverses both sections and reaches the eardrum.

- Expose the ear canal by holding up the ear flap.
- Place the ointment or drops in the ear canal.

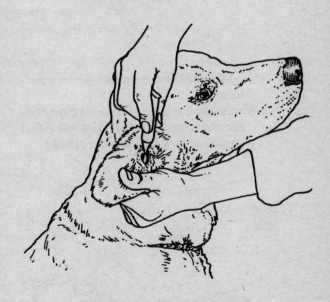

- Massage the ear canal by rubbing the back of the ear where it meets the head. (You may hear a squelch sound. That means that the medicine is making its way down the canal to the ear drum.)

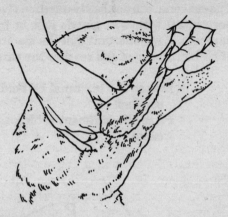

- Try to make the ear squelch for two minutes.
- Wipe away the excess fluid using your finger and a wad of cotton. (Do not insert anything deep into the ear canal.)

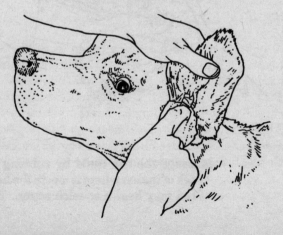

23 Splints, Bandages & Drains

Overview

Splints, bandages and drains are important aids to healing. A splint holds a limb in the correct position so that it can mend. A bandage keeps a wound clean, helps to prevent infection and protects against further injury. A drain is placed in a wound so that excess fluid does not collect. If one of these devices is being used, you should check it often. If you discover any swelling, excessive drainage, foul odors or additional sores, you should contact your veterinarian.

When checking areas of your dog that may be painful, use caution to avoid being injured. If your dog does bite you, seek medical attention.

Splints

A splint is used to position a leg to facilitate the healing of broken bones. It has to be snug enough to hold the limb in the correct position. However, it should not be so tight that it restricts the blood circulation, leads to swelling or causes pressure sores. A splint is difficult to place; most dogs need to be sedated or anesthetized before one can be applied. Caring for one can also be difficult.

Care of a Splint

- Check top and bottom for swelling 3 times a day. Do this by putting your finger in both the top and bottom of the splint.
  - The top of the splint should be snug but you should be able to insert your finger.

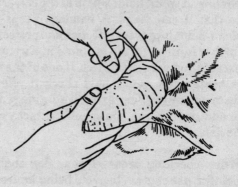

  - You should be able to put your finger in between the toes. They should not be cold or swollen.

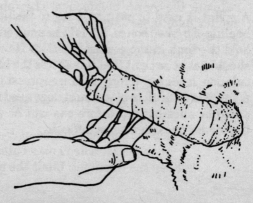

- Check for rubbing and sores 3 times a day.
    - The top of the splint should be able to move slightly when the leg is moved.
    - Your finger should be dry when you pull it out from between the toes. If it is not, there may be open sores draining fluid.
- Keep the dog quiet. Limit the amount of its exercise. Do not let it run free; keep it on a leash.
- Keep the splint clean. Put an old sock over it and tape it in place.
- Keep the splint dry. When going outside, tape a plastic bag or sheet around it. Remove the plastic when going back inside.
- If it chews the splint, put an Elizabethan collar on the dog (see page 159).

Bandages

Bandages help to keep a wound clean and dry, thus reducing the chance of infection. They also protect against additional damage.

Care of a Bandage

- Check for swelling and pus around the wound area. These are signs of infection.
- Keep the bandage clean and dry. Cover it with plastic when going outside.
- Keep the dog quiet. Limit the amount of

exercise. Do not let it run free; keep it on a leash.
- If it chews the bandage, put an Elizabethan collar on the dog (see page 159).

Drains

Drains are devices that allow pus and excess fluid to escape from a wound. This aids the healing process. They occasionally need to be cleaned in order to maintain efficiency. Do not be afraid to work with drains; they rarely hurt the dog when manipulated.

There are two common types of drains. A loop drain is a loop of tape that goes through the skin and is closed with a knot.

A penrose drain is a short piece of very soft plastic tube placed in the wound. One or both ends of the tube protrude from the skin. The fluid drains around the tube, not through it.

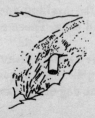

Care of a Drain

- Prepare the drain for cleaning.
    - Loop drains—Pull the knot to the other end of the incision.

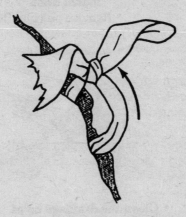

- Penrose drains—Wiggle the end of the drainage tube.

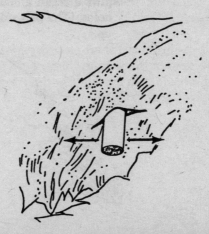

- Remove excess pus and fluid from drainage holes.
    - Soak some gauze with 3% hydrogen peroxide.
    - Dab gauze over drainage holes to loosen dried pus and fluid.
    - Remove pus and fluid.

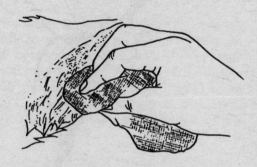

- Clean the drainage holes.
    - Fill eye dropper or syringe with 3% hydrogen peroxide.
    - Squirt a small amount into the holes. (The peroxide will foam up.)

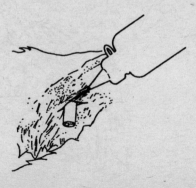

- Dab dry with gauze.
- Repeat 3 times a day or as instructed by your veterinarian.
- If it chews the drain, put an Elizabethan collar on the dog.

Elizabethan Collar

An Elizabethan collar is a large plastic collar that fits around a dog's neck. It is named after a ruffle that people in England used to wear in the time of Queen Elizabeth I. It prevents the dog from pawing at its eyes and ears or from chewing at stitches, sores, splints, bandages and drains. Your veterinarian will give you a collar if your dog needs to wear one.

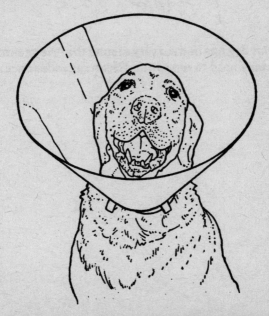

When placing a collar on your dog, fit it just tight enough so that the collar will not slip over the head. Use a strip of gauze to tie it on.

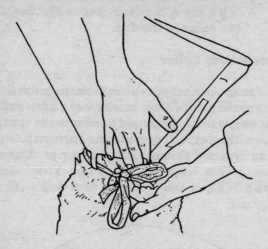

If your dog has had surgery around the face or ears, you may need to remove and clean the collar once a day.

24   Before & After Surgery

Overview

There may be times when it is in your dog's best interest to undergo surgery. In such an instance, there are steps that you can take before and after the operation to help your dog. This chapter gives you some general guidelines. However, some operations require special preparation and care. Your veterinarian will instruct you on the proper action.

BEFORE SURGERY

Preparing Your Dog for Surgery

An operation requires that your dog be given an anesthetic, which exposes it to a slight risk. When anesthetized, a dog loses the protective reflex that closes the windpipe while swallowing. If it were to vomit, a portion may go down the windpipe and into the lungs. This could limit its capacity to breathe and may even result in death. You can help minimize this risk.

What to Do

- No food on the night before surgery.
- No water on the night before surgery. (Very old dogs and those with kidney problems should have access to water throughout the night.)

- If you do feed your dog on the morning of the operation, do NOT hide this fact from the doctor. It is better to delay surgery than to have a serious problem come up while under anesthesia.

AFTER SURGERY

You will need to monitor your dog closely for a couple of weeks. Doing so will help ensure that it is healing properly and without complications.

The First 24 Hours

Most surgery takes place in the morning or early afternoon. The following steps assume that surgery took place then. Your veterinarian will give you instructions on how to care for your dog during the first 24 hours.

- Do not give food or water until the dog is fully awake (usually the morning after surgery). Until then, it will still be under the effects of the anesthesia. Food and water may make it vomit.
- Encourage rest. Keep the dog indoors in a quiet, dark area.
- Do not touch the wound unless instructed to do so.
- Do not be alarmed if the wound bleeds a small amount. (If there is profuse bleeding, call the veterinarian immediately.)

Until the Stitches Come Out

Stitches normally come out 10 to 14 days after the surgery. The stitches that you can see are usually non-dissolvable; your veterinarian will remove them when appropriate. Stitches beneath the skin are usually dissolvable. They will slowly disappear over the course of several weeks.

Until the stitches are taken out or disappear, you should watch your dog carefully. Its activities should be restricted; if not, the wound may open or tear. This could lead to another operation and a longer period of recovery.

- Exercise only on a leash. Do not let it run free or swim.
- Do not clean the wound unless instructed to do so.
- Do not bathe your dog.
- Check the wound every day for swelling. Swelling can be the result of several factors.

    - Reaction to stitches—This is the most common cause. The inflamed area does not diminish in size when pressed. And it is usually not too painful or hot to the touch.

    - Organs or tissue extending through incision—Abdominal surgery requires cutting through all of the muscle layers of the abdomen. Stitches that pull muscle layers together sometimes break down or pull apart, allowing abdominal organs and tissue to poke through and form swelling under the skin. If you push this swelling, it will decrease in size. It usually does not feel hot. If a piece of white abdominal fat extends through the skin, do not pull it out; take your dog to your veterinarian immediately.

• Infection—This is often hot to the touch with a thick creamy-colored discharge. The area usually cannot be reduced in size when pushed unless pus comes out between the stitches.

Contact Your Veterinarian If....

* There is any evidence of infection.
* There is any swelling (unless it is obviously caused by the stitches alone).
* There is anything protruding through the wound.
* There is a high temperature (104 degrees or above).
* The dog is not eating.
* The dog is still very sleepy after 48 hours.
* The dog is vomiting or has diarrhea.

25   Rehabilitation

Overview

Rehabilitation involves the principles ensuring that recovery from an injury or surgery is both complete and as rapid as possible. One of the most important aspects of rehabilitation, giving medication, is discussed in Chapter 22 (see page 165). Rest and gradual increase of activity make up the additional components of a rehabilitation program.

These ideas are simply guidelines. Your veterinarian can recommend the best steps to take that apply to your dog's particular condition.

THE REST PERIOD

Rest requires that the dog's activities be limited. Overexertion during this period can pull stitches, rip bandages, move a splint and strain muscles. This may cause great damage and greatly increase the time needed for recovery. In some cases, aggravated injuries can result in permanent damage.

What to Do

- Confine dog to the home.
- Limit exercise to short walks.
- Keep dog on leash at all times when outside.

AFTER THE REST PERIOD

After the initial healing period, you should increase your dog's daily activities. This should be done gradually; too much exercise soon after a debilitating injury may cause additional damage. This especially applies to dogs that have been wearing splints or other devices that constrict movement. When not used, joints tend to stiffen and muscles may atrophy. There are a few steps that you can take to help your dog resume a normally active life.

Joint Stimulation

A stiff joint lacks synovial fluid, the natural lubrication that aids in smooth movement. You can stimulate the production of this lubricant and begin the process of loosening the joint. You can also start to activate muscles that may have become weak due to lack of use.

What to Do

- Gently move each of the stiff joints in their natural direction.

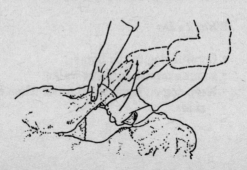

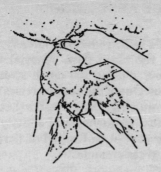

- Use care not to force movement; this can be painful.

Massage

Massage improves the flow of blood and will stimulate atrophied muscles.

What to Do

- Place fingers and thumbs on the muscles to be massaged.
- Gently kneed the muscles.
- Work towards the heart, not away from it.

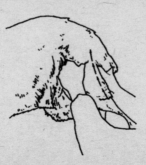

Exercise

Exercise should be introduced gradually. The goal is to activate the blood flow, synovial fluid and muscles without placing too much stress on the joints and bones. One of the best exercises to accomplish this is swimming. Gentle walks that increase both in duration, frequency and activity are also good. Running should be limited at first, but increased as progress is made.

References

Alpo Veterinary Panel for Alpo Pet Center. *Canine Nutrition and Feeding Management.* Allentown, Pennsylvania: Alpo Pet Foods, Inc., 1984.

Animal Medical Center (William J. Kay, DVM, Chief of Staff) with Elizabeth Randolph. *The Complete Book of Dog Health.* New York: Macmillan Publishing Company, 1985.

AVMA Council on Biologic and Therapeutic Agents. "Canine and Feline Immunization Guidelines." *Journal of the American Veterinary Medical Association* (August 1, 1989): 314-317.

Catcott, E.J., DVM, PhD. ed. *Canine Medicine, 4th ed.* Santa Barbara, California: American Veterinary Publications, Inc., 1979.

Ettinger, Stephen J., DVM. *Textbook of Veterinary Internal Medicine: Disease of the Dog and Cat. 2nd ed.* Philadelphia: W.B. Saunders Company, 1983.

Kirk, Robert W., DVM, ed. *Current Veterinary Therapy VIII: Small Animal Practice.* Philadelphia: W. B. Saunders Company, 1983.

Kirk, Robert W., DVM, ed. *Current Veterinary Therapy IX: Small Animal Practice.* Philadelphia: W. B. Saunders Company, 1986.

Kirk, Robert W., DVM, ed. *Current Veterinary Therapy X: Small Animal Practice.* Philadelphia: W. B. Saunders Company, 1989.

Kirk, Robert W. DVM. *First Aid for Pets.* New York: E.P. Dutton, 1978.

Kirk, Robert W., DVM and Stephen I. Bistner, DVM. *Handbook of Veterinary Procedures and Emergency Treatment, 4th ed.* Philadelphia: W. B. Saunders, 1895.

Siegmund, Otto H., et al. eds. *The Merck Veterinary Manual, 5th ed.* Rahway, New Jersey: Merck & Co, Inc., 1979.

Urquhart, G.M., J. Armour, J.L. Duncan, A. M. Dunn and F.W Jennings. *Veterinary Parasitology.* New York: Churchill Livingstone, Inc., 1987.

Index